*How Will You
Feel Tomorrow?*

How Will You Feel Tomorrow?

NEW WAYS TO PREDICT ILLNESS

Samuel Silverman, M.D.

STEIN AND DAY/*Publishers*/New York

First published in 1973
Copyright © Samuel Silverman 1973
Library of Congress Catalog Card No. 73-82111
All rights reserved
Designed by David Miller
Printed in the United States of America
Stein and Day/*Publishers*/Scarborough House, Briarcliff Manor, N.Y. 10510
ISBN 0-8128-1635-8

1775913

Contents

5

Contents

Contents

Contents

PART THREE: *Some Applications of Psychological Prediction*

Unhealthy weight fluctuation can be foretold and dealt with early by looking for such clues as food love, a need to look "unappetizing," "oral dreams," and preoccupation with the eating problems of others.

Not if you heed such emotional signals as apathy instead of interest, a need to escape from internal conflicts, and difficulties in adapting to the unfamiliar.

These result from spasms, hormonal and nervous system disturbances which often can be anticipated from the psychological signs spelled out in this chapter.

PART FOUR: *Forecasting the Outcome of Illness*

Contents

PART FIVE: New Preventive Measures

Preface

How can you tell if your health is in danger? Pain, fever, lumps, persistent cough, unusual weight loss, recurrent bleeding, are some of the familiar signals (not always heeded) that you need a prompt medical checkup. But are you aware that emotion is also a source of warnings that all is not well with your body? My purpose in writing this book is to demonstrate this, to help you recognize when psychological clues *predict* the likelihood of physical disease.

I discovered these clues during an in-depth psychological study of patients. The subjects were not physically sick when they first came to my attention. I found that their emotions not only signaled the likelihood of bodily disturbances, but also indicated what part of the body would be affected, often before physical manifestations or even the most sophisticated laboratory tests did so.

Thus, the book deals with predictors—not causes—of illness. Are you aware of the many disguised forms in which emotional stress warns us our health is in jeopardy? Do you know when exposure to stress does *not* signal physical disease? Are you aware that its accuracy as predictor increases when other psychological clues are also present?

It is impossible within the scope of this book to give examples of psychological predictors in all bodily disorders. I have tried to select, for detailed consideration, some conditions that affect many persons. Discussed are *specific emotional signals* which by themselves can warn of cancer, heart

11

disease, weight disturbances, sickness during vacations, physical complications in sexual life, developing infections, and dental problems.

There is a further use to which you can put psychological predictors—different ones—and that is when you are already sick and certain vital questions confront you. Will you get worse? Will the illness be drawn out? How will you respond to medication, to surgery?

Most of the cases are drawn from my clinical practice. Some are unusual. However, the psychological predictors I describe are applicable to all persons—even though their personalities are less complicated, their emotional problems less troublesome, and their physical ailments less severe. Knowing about these warning signals can spare you weeks or months of needless disability and discomfort from illness or its complications. In fact, if as many people learn to recognize the psychological clues as have become familiar with the physical indicators of body illness, we will be well on the way to more effective prevention of untold personal suffering and economic loss.

PART ONE

*Conflict
and
Prediction
of
Illness*

1

Three Uptight People

THE EYES HAVE IT

Belvedere was looking forward to a date with one of the coeds in his course. It was well known around campus that the middle-aged, nearsighted professor and his wife had not been getting along. They always had been incompatible, but after their children had married and left, the situation had become intolerable. Belvedere, quick to admire a shapely figure, now found himself more preoccupied than ever with any beautiful girl who signed up for his lectures. One of them in particular attracted him; and she, although recently married, played a flirtatious game. They met secretly several times to talk and plan for the occasion when they could be more intimate. Such an opportunity occurred when the girl's husband became ill and had to be hospitalized.

A few nights later she and Belvedere went to a motel some miles away, registering as a couple under a false name. They planned to remain only a few hours. Intense lovemaking took place. The professor found himself staring in fascination at his partner's beautiful body, examining every curve, nook, and orifice. He had placed a mirror nearby and left the light on so that he could watch the action. He had to raise his head rather sharply to see this in the mirror, and noted vaguely in his excitement that the electric bulb was shining directly into his eyes.

The next morning in class, Belvedere saw light flashes every time he moved his head. Later, when a murkiness

15

began to cloud his vision, he became alarmed and consulted an eye specialist. He was stunned by the doctor's finding that an immediate operation was necessary to save him from blindness. He was suffering from a detached retina—in both of his eyes. Many people with this trouble are myopic, are middle-aged or older, have had a previous eye injury or surgery, or have suffered from diabetes. Belvedere was middle-aged and myopic, but had had no eye injuries and was not diabetic. Could the disorder have been predicted? Yes. It practically had been, as you shall see later.

EMOTIONS SIGNAL BODILY DISEASE

Even if you have noted that physical responses are influenced by your moods, you may find it hard to believe that there was any predictable connection between the professor's escapade and his eye problem. Yet I will soon describe some equally surprising cases in which illness could have been forecast from psychological clues long before it occurred. The main reason for presenting such clinical material and for writing this book is to explain how emotions provide guidelines that help you recognize when you and your family are apt to become physically ill, what your reactions to becoming ill may be, and when conflict is likely to complicate your recovery from disease. These guidelines are in the form of specific psychological clues, new additions to the physical warning signals of illness with which you are probably at least somewhat familiar. But before going on to the next case, let's take a brief look at some basics.

When minor physical reactions associated with stress persist and become troublesome, we may consult a physician. If he diagnoses nervous tension, he will seldom explore its source and cause. Instead, he will usually give us some quick reassurance and a prescription for tranquilizers. This may or may not be helpful. Unfortunately, there may be more to our psychological disturbance than is apparent. What many of us don't realize—and too often neither do our physicians —is that our emotional upset could be the first signal of impending bodily disease—acute, chronic, perhaps disabling, even fatal.

Thus one reason it is so vital to know more about how hangups affect our bodies is that we can then teach ourselves to watch for times when we are under a strain; this, in turn, will enable us to be on the lookout for the very earliest signs that conflict is beginning to attack our bodies. But this is only part of the story. Knowing more about psychological predictors can help us in another way; we can thereby become more aware of how our feelings—not only before, but *after* we become physically ill—may complicate, prolong, or in other ways interfere with recovery. If, for example, we are apathetic, uninterested in what's going on around us, this is a sign that our emotions are blocked from expression, which may add to the burdens of an already malfunctioning body. Recognizing and relieving such an emotional state can help us to get better faster.

Another sig .al that convalescence will be slow is a seeming contentment with being ill. It indicates that certain needs —to be cared for, to be relieved of responsibilities, to be forgiven for our sins—are in part satisfied by being sick. But perhaps we can find some better way to gratify them. Other unexpected troubles are apt to occur when we take drugs for illness or discomfort of any kind. If a doctor prescribes the medicine, his competence and experience safeguard us to an extent against undesirable side effects. Nevertheless, these may still occur. The usual explanation is that they are caused by unforeseen biochemical or physiological factors. That may be so. However, when conflicts trouble us, further disruption of our physiology occurs and our reactions to drugs are then especially apt to go

17

askew. There are psychological signs that predict this. A doctor who is familiar with these as well as with our physical condition is better able to choose when and what to prescribe, and thus can reduce untoward effects from medication.

But many people, driven by hangups and perhaps physical needs, take drugs on their own—tranquilizers, sedatives, amphetamines, alcohol, marijuana, hashish, heroin, and others. These self-administered drugs, especially in the presence of great emotional tension, can so disturb your perceptions, mood, and judgment that you will act in ways that endanger your health.

DIRTY-NEEDLE DISEASE

For example, another true story is that of Fawn, who was eighteen when she entered college. Her grades in her small-town high school had been tops, but at the big-city college she found herself a small fish in a big pond. She had difficulty making friends because many of her classmates seemed too uninhibited and too radical, and she was miserably lonely. On a visit home for Thanksgiving, she blurted out her unhappiness to her parents, who enraged her by warning that she should stick to her schoolwork and forget about having fun. After an emotional storm in which she and her parents screamed at each other, she cut her visit short and returned to school.

An abrupt change occurred in Fawn. Almost overnight she became uninhibited and began to sleep around. She smoked pot and experimented with acid; she even shot heroin one night. Her schoolwork suffered, until finally the midyear examinations loomed before her. She tried desperately to prepare for them but felt tired and feverish, ached all over, and had no appetite. One morning she awoke after a troubled sleep and on looking in the mirror saw her face had turned yellow.

Again, it may be hard to believe there was any connection between Fawn's changed behavior and the serious illness —viral hepatitis—that befell her. Or that it could have been predicted. Later I'll explain how and why this would have been possible. But first, it is important to realize that for years—indeed for centuries—we have not fully understood illness because we've been stuck on the question of whether it is emotionally *or* physically caused. Even though the best thinking today considers disease to be caused by the interaction of a number of things, physical signs, symptoms, and laboratory tests continue to be regarded as the prime, if not exclusive, indicators of bodily disorder. That's because, hitherto, psychological clues have not been specific enough to be useful for this purpose. Now such clues have been discovered.

CANCER ALERT

Take the case of Losgroth, fifty-five years old and in good health, a successful politician holding an office of some importance. He and his wife lived quietly and simply. His integrity and reputation were unquestioned; his constituents called him "Mr. Incorruptible." Now he was being considered as his party's nominee for very high office and was engaged in an unusually energetic campaign prior to the nominating convention. He was the favorite in a field of three contenders. As the campaign progressed, his expectations ran high.

But at the convention, unexpectedly, behind-the-scenes maneuvering began to turn the odds against him. Deals were made, and one of his opponents suddenly and dramatically carried the convention.

For a few weeks afterward Losgroth appeared stunned and not his usual self. Then he seemed to recover his equanimity, apparently determined to give his best in finishing out his term. Only he knew what a terrible emotional upset he had experienced and what an incredible effort he had made to push it out of his mind. He had not heeded these physical warnings of impending trouble and had kept them secret. But his wife noticed that he looked thinner and somewhat pale. Though she urged him to have a checkup, he refused. Meanwhile his successful rival at the convention went on to win the election. At the end of his term of office, Losgroth announced his retirement from public service and began to consider several lucrative job offers in private industry. He finlly chose one, but before he could begin his new work he developed a persistent, severe back pain. This finally drove him to see his physician, who recommended hospitalization for futher tests. X rays showed a suspicious spot in his spine that the doctors thought was metastatic cancer-spread there from some other part of his body.

Is it fair to say—that this sequence of events is proof that psychological signs are the first warnigns of disease? Or is the study of cells and hormones the only way of anticipating Losgroth's ailment, and should we therefore discount his shattering emotional experience?

Each viewpoint is too narrowly extreme and simplistic to explain by itself how the complex process of human illness can be predicted. Modern medicine had discovered that harmful psychological factors *always* precede an illness—if the physician takes the trouble to listen carefully to the patient. But it's complicated. For instance, not everyone exposed to stress necessarily comes down with a disease. Some people do *not* become ill, and do *not* die, even after terrible emotional experiences. They have an unusual capacity for coping with the great strain they're under, or are fortunate enough then to be exposed quickly to more favorable life situations (or both). Some people develop mental disorders. They deal, unsuccessfully, with their problems through psychological channels, and even mitigating situational experience may be insufficient to relieve their conflicts. Others act nervous or have a minor physical disorder for a while and then get over it; the extent of their disturbance seems to be limited. Here again, unsuspected psychological strengths or favorable life circumstances may be operating. Apart from emotions, heredity and other factors—social, economic, cultural, and political—are involved. So it's not at all a simple matter to determine exactly what goes on in our emotions *and* bodies to make one of us escape illness, another become a little depressed or suffer some mild indispostion, and still another develop a serious and perhaps fatal disease. However, there are psychological guidelines that people can use to understand better what their chances of becoming physically ill may be.

WHICH TARGET ORGAN?

Professor Belvedere, Fawn, and Losgroth were all suffering from emotional conflicts. Why did one develop an eye problem, another have liver trouble, and the third, lung cancer? Could the target organ in each instance have been predicted?

A partial answer can be put very simply by saying that each of us has a particular set of psychological and physical safety valves for inner tension. We speak our mind, become depressed, have daydreams, act violently, run to the toilet, get a headache, or drain off tension in other ways. However, should stress become severe, our psychological safety valves may break down and then we suffer from severe mental disorders; or these outlets are bypassed and then the burden of dealing with stress falls on our bodies. That's when we become susceptible to physical disease. When illness actually strikes, it doesn't do so randomly, but at vulnerable spots in our bodies unique for each of us. Hereditary factors influence what our particular vulnerability will be—but, in addition, a major determinant is our emotional state, especially during our childhood illnesses. Any tensions occurring then will become linked with our physical condition, with the afflicted organ or organ system—which becomes "sensitized." It's as if thereafter these body parts were especially susceptible to malfunction when we are exposed again to emotional strain.

How then, later on, before illness strikes, can we tell what kind it's apt to be? Or its site? Not by pigeonholing ourselves into so-called personality types, popular though that discredited concept continues to be. Instead, the following may be very early clues: (1) a history of previous disturbances in a particular body area, preceded or accompanied by emotional upset, e.g., stomach trouble (nausea, vomiting, indigestion) and anger at parents; the sensitized organ is the stomach and will likely malfunction again during subsequent stress; (2) awareness in ourselves of persistent physical sensations, discomfort, or symptoms similar to those of a sick person with whom we are or have been emotionally involved; (3) frequently dreams whose symbolic manifestations or latent content indicate unusual preoccupation with a particular part of the body or a particular physical function.

Take Professor Belvedere, alone with his thoughts as he waited to be wheeled into the operating room. He tried to tell himself this operation could not be happening, that only a month before he had had an eye checkup and nothing had been found. But he knew he was leaving things out—he had been warned earlier when he first had gone to see his family doctor about his aching eyes. At that time he had had an unnerving talk about his cold, sick marriage. And about his sex life. From childhood on, he confessed, he had been a voyeur. Sex and looking had become incredibly entangled. The sight of a woman's body—even partly undressed —of love play, of intercourse itself, had a powerful, arousing effect, either when he just thought about it or in reality. Every time he felt tense or depressed he would look—into other people's houses and bedrooms, at pornographic books, movies, burlesque, and sex exhibitions. But discreetly. No one ever knew or suspected. It had become his escape from marital or professional problems, from almost everything that bothered him. Look and get sexually excited, even to ejaculation, so he could have some relief from tension. But it never worked out that way. He always feared he would be caught and shamed, and afterward his eyes would ache. His father, in his old age, had developed cataracts and become a pathetic hypochondriac. Belvedere, who still felt terribly guilty about wanting to be rid of him, then became concerned that he would get the same disability, whenever his own eyes hurt. This physical identification with his father was another clue to what part of Belvedere's body would be particularly vulnerable to illness.

Marriage turned out to be a disaster. His wife, a former beauty queen, was selfish and cold, insisting on darkness and concealment during their physical intimacy—what there was of it. None of his academic successes could make up for the frustrating nights when he tossed restlessly in bed—as he had done so often during childhood.

Each year more layers of anxiety, hatred, and guilt had piled up. Unknown to Belvedere, the stage had been set. There is only so much strain anyone can take before mind or body begins to break down. And his eyes were prime targets. Their normal functioning had become associated with forbidden sexual impulses, anger, and expectation of punishment. He became very frightened when he began to have recurrent dreams of being lost and unable to find his way. This was still another clue that he would have trouble with his eyesight.

His family doctor had warned him, "Your way of dealing with tension isn't doing you any good. You've got problems which need expert help—otherwise something's going to give way." Well, the doctor had been right—even though Belvedere never thought, and maybe his doctor never thought, specifically of his eyes. Something *had* given way because, despite the warning, Belvedere had done nothing to relieve the enormous strain he was under. Instead he tried to forget it.

When we cannot cope with our inner conflicts by psychological means (fantasies, feelings, or behavior), and don't get relief through favorable life circumstances or treatment, our bodies catch the impact of the strain we're under. This is especially true if certain parts of them have been conditioned to react in this way when we've been emotionally upset in the past.

If we go back to Fawn, her fatigue and malaise during the weeks preceding her illness were connected in her thoughts and dreams with expectations of becoming a chronic invalid. Her mother for many years had been ill and too concerned with her own gall bladder trouble to give her daughter much attention—except to take her to the doctor from time to time. The doctor said that Fawn, like her mother, had an irritable digestive system (a comparison which made a deep but hidden impression on her), and regularly gave her injections for what he called her "poor blood." Those visits were big productions, with the screaming child being held down while she was jabbed in the arm or behind with what looked to her like an enormous needle. The doctor did not recognize any connection between her feelings of deprivation and her bodily ailments. But her digestive system was becoming sensitized to act up whenever Fawn felt particularly neglected or rejected.

What about Losgroth? In the hospital he was a model patient. He had gone through an array of tests, laboratory studies, and other procedures that would have driven anyone else up a wall, but he bore them stoically. Even with the gravity of his physical condition increasing, with the doctors unable to find the original location of the cancer that had spread to his spine, Losgroth remained outwardly impassive. But late at night, he found it hard to fall asleep in his quiet, private room, despite sedation. During those lonely hours he thought a great deal about his past, as he had been doing for several months now. And what had preoccupied him? His father, that remarkably successful lawyer who treated him like an expensive toy. A hulk of a man who had asthma and died in a plane crash when Losgroth was twelve years old. And what about his mother? His thoughts became blurred. He dozed fitfully as troublesome dreams about his wheezing father whom he had loved and hated disturbed his sleep. When he awoke he kept thinking about the two severe attacks of pneumonia he himself had had while mourning his father's sudden death. All this he had hidden. But now the façade of imperturbability had barely been maintained. Unfamiliar tears trickled down his face. It was dark; he was alone; and no one would know that the man of logic had feelings.

After one of many consultations, a doctor lingered by Losgroth's bedside, and for once Losgroth let himself go and talked openly. And for the first time since his childhood, Losgroth cried in front of another person. He spoke of those incredibly difficult early years when he had been surrounded by every material advantage and a succession of nursemaids, but deprived of a single friendly, warm heart. In this sudden flow of words and intimacy he unexpectedly even remembered things about his mother. It came to him in a flash that when he was only five, he had been told by a servant that his mother had died shortly after he was born. His innocent child's mind had taken that to mean it was *his* fault that she had died. Later he heard that her death was due to a brain tumor, but it made no difference. His guilt, his feelings of deprivation, his hatred, practically all his emotions, had become walled off. He developed into a coldly logical, controlled, moralistic being . . . Now as he talked on, he was experiencing something strange. Was it a feeling of human warmth—in himself, in the compassionate listener? Was it the beginning of an inner peace at long last? The doctor promised to come back the next day, but by then Losgroth had slipped into a coma.

Terrible tensions had been tearing Losgroth apart for three months without any chance for skillful intervention to relieve them. Yet he had desperately needed help. Critical stress had upset the psychological balance of many years. Now enormous energies were being released and had nowhere to go but against his body, disrupting its normal processes. And what was the target area? Hidden in one of the main passageways to his right lung was a nub of cancer tissue, too small to be picked up by X rays or other physical tests. And it was sending its deadly offshoots to his spine.

GUILT AND PHYSICAL AILMENTS

The mind-body relationship was known in a crude way in antiquity. But primitive man believed that his ailments were caused by malignant spirits whose displeasure he had incurred. These supernatural beings were representations of his conscience. He tried to anticipate their malevolence toward him. This he did by examining the entrails of sacrificial animals, looking for omens that he might become ill. Later it was thought that immorality was a sign that you would become ill—either physically or mentally—and when you did, it was considered a punishment for your offenses.

These early recognitions that mental disturbance—particularly guilt—in some way signaled physical illness were crude, simplistic expressions of what I refer to as unconscious conflicts heralding bodily disorder. Today we know that the "unconscious" is a complex of mental activities outside awareness. It includes thoughts concerned with our sexual or hostile impulses and the defenses against them as well as the workings of our conscience. Often we are aware only vaguely that psychological defenses or a conscience (which may be very strict) exist in us. The latter works in such a subtle and hidden fashion that it can even contribute to our hurting ourselves needlessly or developing a bodily ailment without our being aware of the connection. This is how Belvedere's conscience had been doing him in. All the while he *thought* he was getting his kicks out of sex shows (and it was an inadequate erotic release anyway), another part of his mind never stopped condemning him for this looking. Partly he was aware of this from the guilt he felt; partly he suffered from aching eyes, which had come to represent organs of wickedness as well as of sexual pleasure in his unconscious. But at the time of the motel incident an ominous change had occurred. Belvedere seemed no longer troubled by guilt feelings, though he continued to give in to his erotic impulses. It was a signal that his body would suffer much more.

Fawn, miserably lonely at college, had thrown herself into a whirl of new experiences, especially those that she had formerly considered bad, trying to put aside feelings of not belonging. A surge of rebelliousness, released by the quarrel with her parents, helped overcome—though only temporarily—the prohibitions of her conscience. What did she care if she did wrong? It got her instant friends. Her frenetic activity, her air of independence, masked but did not eliminate her dependent feelings. Like many adolescents Fawn had sought relief from inner turmoil in these ways. As time went on, something else, unknown to her, forced her further into the mess. It was a need to atone for the guilt that was building up in her despite her defiant behavior. How atone? By exposing herself to situations which had the potential of hurting her—psychologically or physically. The voice of caution in her had become stilled in more ways than one, especially after she got into the drug scene. Though it had terrified her and she hadn't wanted to use heroin, she didn't want to lose her new friends by being chicken either. The subsequent illness from the unsterile needle came to represent a symbolic punishment. And ironically,

27

as if the misery of being so sick weren't enough, she kept being pricked by needles (shining, sterile ones) in the hospital. Though they were now being used to take blood samples to follow the course of her recovery, she could not shake her childhood fear of them.

Fawn's disturbed actions (disguised expressions of her fight with her conscience) were warnings that she was exposing herself to physical risks and could get hurt. And it had come true.

There are plenty of people whose emotion is walled off and who are not troubled by any symptoms of tension. However, if you are such a person and your emotional equilibrium is sufficiently shaken by stress or other factors, it will begin to crumble, and then disturbing thoughts and feelings may become conscious and indicate the presence of great strain. Because these are often very early indicators of developing illness, keeping them secret may put your emotional *and* physical well being in jeopardy.

Losgroth had been conditioned from childhood to be secretive about himself. As a youngster his chief contacts were with a succession of impersonal governesses. So as he was growing up, he had learned to keep his feelings to himself and to think as objectively as he could. While still a youngster, an ambition whose true meaning was unknown to him began to burn in his mind—a craving for power. A strict conscience drove him to seek perfection in everything he did. After college and a brief try at business, he had entered politics and had experienced success after success until that defeat at the nominating convention—that incredibly painful defeat that had shattered him and ended his political career. Who could have guessed from his outward demeanor and conversation that he had been profoundly disturbed? Only he knew that he had failed in his attempt to outdo his father and hence felt a complete failure. He tried to stifle a tremendous rage against those who conspired to defeat him, and he could not bear the pressure that kept building in his chest.

ONE SHIED; ONE TRIED; ONE DIED

After Belvedere had had his eye operation, he was told it was not altogether successful. His vision would be impaired, and there was still danger of blindness. This was confirmed by a number of consultants. Bitterly disappointed and let down, Belvedere, who had already renounced psychiatric help, now turned away from the whole field of medicine. Despite his education and sophistication he began in his desperation to search for any possibility of cure—no matter how far-fetched. And that's how he came to Dr. Duckrie and his cosmometric machine. It was an awesome-looking apparatus, with its flashing lights and many dials. As Duckrie, who was not a medical doctor, explained: "It harnesses cosmic rays and directs their healing effect in the proper strength against the diseased body parts."

When we are seriously ill or badly disabled and the best medical treatment is getting nowhere or is unavailable, the need for some relief may become irresistible. At such times we may overlook objective psychological clues that indicate an urgent need for relief of accompanying tensions by reliable therapy and, instead, reach out for any ray of hope. Superstition, trickery, and miracle-mongering (often in the respectable guise of faith) stand ready to offer such hope. This has been true for hundreds of years. Being in a place famous for its curative powers allows suggestible people to imagine that an omnipotent, invisible force can have a similar healing effect on them. The more believers that are gathered together, the more each individual's faith is reinforced. It is a fact that some illnesses (chiefly those classified as hysterical) often show some improvement under such circumstances, but complete cures have not been verified. So although faith healing shouldn't be dismissed entirely, relying on faith alone to cure or alleviate illness is hit-or-miss, even foolhardy if it makes you bypass available medical (and psychological) care.

Poor Belvedere might have escaped the tragic consequences of his hangups if he had followed through on his family doctor's advice when the latter recognized some of the psychological signs that illness was imminent. After the unsuccessful operation, emotional indicators revealed that he needed competent help all the more to deal with his inner turmoil and failing sight. Instead, he again ignored his hangups and their signals that his recovery would be complicated. He chose a quack—so his tensions were never released, his eyes got worse, and his case became hopeless.

And where had Fawn turned when she became so upset? Her longing to be cared for and loved was an old need. And there was something else. Like many adolescents, she wanted to experience a sense of freedom from the ties that bound her to her family. She was ready to try new things, especially those that would prove how far she had been liberated from her square parents. But none of it had helped—underneath she was still starved for affection. That her recovery from hepatitis would be slowed up was signaled by her continuing but marked depression. A person who is sick and also suffers from disguised mood disturbances often has a complicated and protracted convalescence because these emotions interfere with the body's recuperative powers. Fawn was unaware of her underlying depression.

But perhaps just because Fawn was still looking for someone who would recognize her needs and because she *was* willing to try new things, she was lucky. For she agreed to see a psychiatrist when her problems, like Professor Belvedere's, were found to go beyond those of the body. And the therapy progressed, aided by a quick, positive doctor-patient relationship. Fawn began to understand how far back into the past her feelings of deprivation extended. And how much rage she still had toward her family, even though it had gone under cover. The treatment gradually taught her how she had expressed her bitter anger in her changed, reckless behavior, in doing all the things that her parents would object to and that would make them unhappy. And she also learned that underneath the reckless fun, her troubled conscience that had pushed her toward the dirty needle and illness was still bothering her. So, though her physical and emotional recovery was slow, she had at least turned away from further disasters, and her future was a lot brighter than the more sophisticated Professor Belvedere's.

But this brings us back to the unfortunate Losgroth, who pretended—and tried to make others (including his doctors) believe—that he was free of emotion. Losgroth had done himself a disservice. If only he had shared his secret, his angry feelings that the convention defeat had been like a mortal blow. If only his wife, his relatives, his doctor, had known earlier that he felt so distraught. He could have been examined immediately and a careful check could have been kept on his physical *and emotional* condition during those three critical months. Helpful psychological clues might have come to light, and the previous link between his attacks of pneumonia and stress (father's death) would have suggested the lung as a target organ. The disease might have been detected before it spread, or it might even have been prevented from developing if the tension that wracked him had been relieved by psychotherapy in conjunction with other medical means. Losgroth's way—his stoicism, his need to present himself as invincible—had worked against him on this occasion and after he was hospitalized. The best physicians were racing against time trying to find the primary site of the cancer. In vain. It would not be discovered until the autopsy. Losgroth was dying.

We see that Belvedere, Fawn, and Losgroth each had

a different attitude toward talking about their conflicts, and this was an important factor in the outcome of their sickness. Belvedere shied away from help, finally distrusted all physicians, and wound up with a quack and impending blindness. Physically sick and depressed, Fawn tried psychotherapy and eventually gained a better understanding of herself as she recovered from her illness. Losgroth died just as he became able to reveal the intense feelings that had been bottled up in him.

Sickness is often not so serious. But you can still spare yourself days or weeks of needless incapacity and discomfort through illness. How? By knowing about these clues and being alerted by them to seek appropriate help early.

Even when there are signs during sickness that emotional factors are influencing its course, formal psychotherapy is often not necessary or even desirable. Support, reassurance, and a chance to release pent-up feelings are sufficient to bring relief from interfering tensions in many instances. This can be done by those caring for you, whether they be doctors, nurses, aides, relatives, or friends, provided they can see you as more than just a stomach, heart, or other organ which isn't working properly, and are aware of the signs that emotional disturbance is interfering with recovery. But when *major* psychological upsets occur during an illness, they must be considered danger signals. They foretell slow healing or possibly death, even when the best medical procedures are being carried out. Under such circumstances, skilled psychiatric help becomes essential.

PART TWO

Prophetic Emotions

2

A New DEW Line Against Disease

How can we tell if illness awaits us? A lump, unusual pain, bleeding, loss of weight—we have been educated to know the meaning of these warnings. We have been conditioned to react to them as red alerts. They are, of course, supplemented by a host of X rays and laboratory tests. Are there any other signals? Yes, and they may be even earlier indicators of impending trouble. But how many of us have been taught to be aware of their presence and significance? Very few of us as yet know that specific psychological clues can help forecast not only the development of a new disease, but also the return or worsening of an old or chronic one. These indicators and their physical counterparts are our distant early warning (DEW) line against attack from bodily illness.

TEN PREDICTORS

You may have read or heard superficial and oversimplified reports about a few psychological clues, but the majority hitherto have not been described in popular articles, and in only one instance in the scientific literature—in a book I wrote on the subject for health professionals.* It is my

*Psychological Clues in Forecasting Physical Illness. New York: Appleton-Century-Crofts, 1970.

35

purpose now to provide you with a thorough and scientific understanding of *all* these clues so that you may have a better idea of when your health is threatened and when it is not. At this point, I will only list the clues and give a brief account of their significance, but I intend to discuss each of them in detail in subsequent chapters.

(1) Recent exposure to stress.

(2) Previous episodes of physical disease, rather than emotional illness, when under a strain.

(3) History of bodily ailments occurring in family members subjected to stress.

(4) A strong tendency to deny unpleasant realities.

(5) Inadequacy of the usual psychological outlets (thoughts, feelings, behavior), especially as tension builds.

(6) Intense rage, pent up or explosively discharged, whose meaning is repressed.

(7) Remorse or self-destructive actions which at first are noticeable and then suddenly disappear without apparent reason.

(8) Repetitive dreams about physical sensations and bodily changes.

(9) Persistent thoughts about symptoms and illnesses of people important to us.

(10) Behavior that could lead us unwittingly to injury or sickness.

RESEARCH PROOF

My own interest in this began as a result of observations made on men and women, all of whom were physically well, who had come to me for analysis. But as I came to know them over a period of time, I noticed that they occasionally developed bodily disorders after an emotional crisis. I began to search back through my notes, and in every instance I discovered that I had written things the patients had said, their feelings and behavior—which had appeared insignificant as signs of impending illness at the time, but which in retrospect seemed to be extraordinarily prophetic. In all cases I discovered that though neither they nor I had realized it when it was happening, they themselves had given ample psychological indication that they were about to come down with a physical illness.

For example, one of my patients had a rip-roaring fight with her mother, who shortly afterward left for an extended world cruise. The patient knew this trip had been scheduled long before, but she kept being plagued by fears that she had lost her mother and would never see her again. For a while the strain she was under and her remorse were painfully evident—and then disappeared. She became almost bland and spoke mostly of trivialities except for two striking dreams. In one she was alone on an ice floe, her body stiff and frozen, floating down an endless river. In the other she was on a rack being tortured by someone she could not see. Except for some references to the coldness of the world and the frailty of the human body, her associations to the dreams dwindled away. A week after her mother's departure, the patient came down with pneumonia. In retrospect I could see that there had been signs of impending illness. The patient had gone through a period of intense stress. Her feelings had then become blocked off—especially her hostility and guilt. Her sleep had been troubled by dreams of loneliness and bodily suffering. I already knew the patient's childhood had been marked by frequent sore throats and colds—those were the only times her mother paid her some attention. An old pattern of response to stress had been stirred up.

After a while I found that many of my patients presented generally similar psychological clues before they became ill. This led me to consider the possibility that such indicators had predictive value—that is, that I could study what my patients said and did with an eye to picking up signals of illness. I tested my theory by noting when particular clusters of these psychological indicators would appear, and then I would predict (to myself) that an illness was imminent. I made this prediction *before* any physical symptoms had become apparent. Sometimes, unexpected ego-boosting or guilt-relieving events lessened tension and its ill effect on the body—and so changed the outcome (away from illness), thus nullifying my predictions. However, in a high percentage of cases my forecast was correct. I also discovered that it was possible to bring out these clues in patients who were in less intensive treatment. In fact, if looked for, the psychological indicators usually can be elicited when a careful history is taken during a medical checkup. And you can learn to detect them yourself. Here are some simple guidelines.

Exposure to stress should always alert us to the possibility of an immediate or later reaction in our bodies. However, if there are no other signs—psychological or physical—it's unlikely that we will become sick. Sometimes stress is disguised and we are not aware of it. But other psychological signs may be present. For instance, suppose we notice that a sense of remorse that's been troubling us disappears. We don't know why, but feel momentarily relieved. The chances are that our emotional balance has undergone a sharp change, one that could have a physical impact. We'd do well then to look carefully at our feelings. Are we holding them back? Are we at least dimly aware that we've tended to bury our emotions? In particular, we ought to be alert to the presence of pent-up rage. Perhaps we've had some troublesome dreams about our bodies or about bodily sensations. All these self-observations may then lead us to the realization that we've been under a strain because of frustration, disappointment, loss, etc., or because anniversaries of such experiences have stirred up conflict in us. A cluster of such signs is a warning that our health may suffer. At this point we can try to recollect how we reacted in the past to stressful events. Were we emotionally upset or did we develop a physical ailment? In addition, let's think of whether our hereditary background indicates we have bodily areas that could be particularly vulnerable. Also, have we been preoccupied with the illnesses of people close to us? The answers to these questions point to the kinds and sites of disease we might possibly develop. Any accompanying physical symptoms or signs we note lend even greater weight to these warnings.

IGNORING HEARTFELT EMOTIONS

The trouble has been that we (and too often our doctors) have not been aware that there are such *specific* psychological warnings. We have focused on physical signs, symptoms, and laboratory tests. While these provide us with valuable information about our health, they often do so relatively late in the development of disease. Specific psychological indicators can alert us much earlier to the likelihood of illness or its recurrence. Then, even if you don't have gross bodily manifestations, it would still be wise to have not only your physical but also your emotional state checked over. That makes it possible to institute appropriate preventive or treatment measures—including modification of tension—at the earliest possible time.

For instance, consider Canboy's case. Before he had his first coronary, he had been climbing the corporate ladder at a dizzying pace. He had had regular medical checkups, which had been "negative." But nobody, including himself, had paid any attention to his thoughts and feelings. If these had been carefully examined, they would have revealed severe tension concealed by frenetic activity, wheeling and dealing, and attempts at outright denial that he was upset. There also could have been noted a long-standing tendency toward moodiness which had strangely disappeared a month before he had been struck down by the coronary. He recovered from the illness seemingly without serious complication and went on to become president of a vast industrial empire.

Once in his life his inner self had surfaced briefly. That was when Canboy, caught in a prolonged moody spell while a student at business school, had a long talk with a psychiatrist. He revealed how a sense of being inferior, not liked, and unwanted had haunted him since childhood. This was behind his need to drive to the top. Even as a child he felt impelled to be better than his father, an inept man. His mother was the strong one in the family. Though Canboy felt neglected by her, he identified strongly with her tenacious drive to overcome all difficulties. As he was growing up, he was subject to temper tantrums, and it took much effort to control them. Frustrations tended to depress him, but he usually worked his way out of them—by devoting all his energies to whatever he was doing.

That one visit to the psychiatrist had opened up too many unpleasant memories. Canboy decided to go no more and not to think again about the pain of his past. Work and more work was the answer—for him. When he married, it was with the understanding that he would be president at work and his wife president at home. Sex was incidental and mechanical. Getting to the top careerwise and socially was their common bond.

As president, Canboy embarked on a program of developing subsidiaries in other countries while retrenching at home—so that many workers were laid off in the domestic plants. To many that seemed reckless and ill advised. But he was not one to brook opposition or interference. As he ruthlessly drove on, implementing his policies, the opposition grew and grew within the great industrial organization and outside it. Then Canboy astonished everyone by announcing his retirement to private life—to peace and freedom from controversy, as he put it. Outwardly he seemed relaxed and content. Inwardly he could not give up his tremendous resentment at actually and secretly having been forced to step down. No one knew, because no one dared ask him, how he really felt, not even his wife and children. Nor his personal physician, an expert in heart disease, but not in emotions.

One day all the media carried the news that Canboy had had a second coronary. Just a week before, he had been given a complete checkup—all negative. At that time his doctors had gone over him inch by inch—physically, that is. But again no questions about his emotional state. If they had gone into that, even though Canboy might have resisted their inquiries, they would have gained some inkling that he again had experienced a sudden, sharp increase in tension. It was approximately the anniversary of his resignation. And painful feelings had been stirred up in him—frustration, a sense of being rejected, bitterness. Most difficult for him was the fact that the new president had continued Canboy's policies, though in a more indirect way, and was encountering no massive opposition. Canboy was infuriated by this. His tremendous need for approval and acclamation grew even greater. His sleep was disturbed by many anxiety dreams.

And then, deceptively, he seemed to become calmer. In reality, his feelings of bitterness and guilt had gone underground. These were all signs that his body would bear the brunt of these pent-up energies. And his heart was the target organ. The precise medical history, the exotic battery of laboratory tests, the EKG, the meticulous physical examination, had revealed nothing at all of Canboy's emotional state and his adaptation to it. So all the psychological indicators which would have pointed to the imminence of a physical breakdown, and would have shown the imperative need for lessening his tension, went by the board.

WARNINGS DURING ILLNESS

And what psychological warnings should we watch for *after* we become sick—warnings that things may go badly for us? Again, you may know in a general way that emotional upset makes recovery more difficult, but here I will list *specifics* for which you should be on the lookout (and discuss them later in detail).

(1) A wholesale denial that anything is wrong.

(2) The opposite—persistent tension and tearfulness.

(3) A buildup of repressed hostility.

(4) Disinterest in people, in reading, listening to the radio, or watching television.

(5) Periods of confusion and apathy. The more we turn our faces to the wall and the more our attitude is one of giving up, the greater the likelihood that our bodies' recuperative powers are being hampered by our emotional conflicts.

Here is an example of what can happen if psychological warning signals before *and* after illness go unheeded. Over a period of six months, Amos had had one bad experience after another. He was refused a promotion at the newspaper where he worked as an assistant editor. His small investment portfolio dwindled to almost nothing in the bear market. He quarreled with his best friend and did not speak to him again. His only child left for a course of study in Europe. Only his wife remained true and faithful by his side, treating him like a king. Amos had been discharged from the Navy during the Korean War because of an ulcer. But it had not bothered him afterward. Now as he began to feel more and more tense, he noted that his digestion was poor, and he diagnosed it as a virus. But the virus didn't go away. Amos kept denying anything was really amiss.

When he received word that his father was ill with cancer of the bowel, Amos showed no emotion. Occasionally the thought flashed through his mind: It serves the s.o.b. right.

Amos had been a battered child, cruelly treated by this father.

Finally, when his stomach pain became unendurable and his vomiting would not stop, he consulted a physician and was hospitalized. A diagnosis of duodenal ulcer with severe obstruction was quickly made, and an operation removing most of his stomach was done. Despite all the tubes and needles that he was hooked up to, despite all the medicines, Amos didn't get better. He couldn't eat, couldn't keep anything down, and lost a lot of weight. His visitors thought he looked like a starved concentration-camp inmate. The surgeons had found an obstructing ulcer, adhesions, and other trouble at the time of operation, but felt they had cleaned it all up. They were puzzled by the complications which were holding back his recovery—the physical complications.

Amos didn't show his feelings to anyone but his wife, and then only in a limited way. Actually he was a seething cauldron of emotions—intense anxiety about his condition, terrible rage at the surgeons and other hospital personnel, who he felt didn't give a hoot about him. Behind all this and hidden even from himself was an incredible guilt about all the dreadful thoughts he had had and was having about his parents—especially his father—about anybody who frustrated his need to be cared for or who hurt him. And this was linked with insidious but ever-growing self-destructive impulses. Amos wouldn't read or look at television. He stared at the wall, trying to shut off all stimuli, especially the disagreeable ones from his body. In effect he was forcing himself into a state of sensory deprivation.

One morning very early he awoke confused, disoriented, insisting he was no longer ill, trying to get out of bed, pulling at tubes and needles. The psychotic episode lasted most of the day and then seemingly was over. Incredibly, this gross danger signal was ignored by his doctors. When friends insisted that Amos see a psychiatrist, he refused.

After some weeks, the surgeons, still focusing on Amos'

physical state and ignoring or not understanding that he was in emotional turmoil, operated again. This time they insisted the trouble had finally been eradicated. But Amos still couldn't keep anything down and his weight dropped even more. The efforts of the surgeons to keep nourishment going into him via a mass of tubes and needles became more frantic. Another brief psychotic episode occurred. Again nothing was done about his emotional state. His wife, deeply troubled, but still tyrannized by the hollow-eyed skeleton, could only go along with the doctors. They were talking about a third operation, but a blood infection set in. When death finally came for Amos, he went not unwillingly.

This is an extreme example of what can happen when signs of emotional upheaval during illness are ignored. However, many less tragic but nevertheless undesirable outcomes may be prevented if some attention is paid to these psychological signs. They warn you of the possibility that apparently endless convalescence, annoying physical complications, and unexpected relapses may interfere with your recovery. In turn, those who care for you during illness will be alerted to the need for relieving your tensions if they know about these indicators.

3

The Hidden Role of Stress

It has become increasingly popular to blame our bodily ills on the environment—and we certainly have good reason to. Bacteria and viruses, polluted air and water, chemicals in our food, noise, extreme weather—all of these are enough to convince us that the world we live in can be hostile. Yet the environmental stress that is most threatening to our physical health is one we are apt to make light of: other people. And we are usually unaware that in each of us there are conflicting emotional forces that are influenced by external events and can then also be very stressful.

It's easy enough to decide we can do without smog or an oil slick on the beach, but how to handle stress from our interactions with other people and from within ourselves is no simple matter. We want and need human companionship and love—so we are often less ready to admit that other people also can be irritants and objects of hatred. The complexity of our emotional makeup and of our human relationships leads to tensions that can be difficult to identify. It is the purpose of this chapter to point out the less obvious forms of psychological stress, and to clarify under what circumstances such stress becomes a useful clue for forecasting disease.

NEED FOR STIMULATION

Not all environmental stress is harmful. In fact, our senses need to be stimulated—we need some nudging and prodding from the outer world if we are to develop normally and remain healthy. This is essential—as part of adequate care—right at the start, in infancy, when a *relatively* happy, relaxed, attentive mother can make all the difference not only in our relationship with her and in our later dealings with others, but also in our physical development. Being fed when hungry, being able to suck enough on a breast or bottle or pacifier, being held firmly yet lovingly, being cuddled and rocked, *and* having our senses stimulated—all satisfy our pleasure needs, help build up our confidence, and favor good health. The least known of these appears to be the need for sensory stimulation: our sense of balance, of being in motion, of being touched and held, as well as our sight and hearing—all have to be sufficiently stimulated for us to develop normally during the first six months of life.

Even abnormal infants—physically handicapped babies—if they are cuddled, held, rocked by the mother, allowed to experience the usual sounds of the household and to move around, are apt to develop personalities not unlike those of normal babies. On the other hand, if a baby without physical handicap is deprived of adequate mothering and his hearing, sight, sense of touch, of balance, of being in motion, are not stimulated enough, he becomes more susceptible to physical illness and may suffer irreversible damage during maturation. While an older child who gets inadequate mothering and sensory stimulation may still develop fairly normally, an infant so neglected during the first six months is in real trouble.

In adulthood, also, to be deprived of environmental stimulation can lead to psychological and bodily disorders. This has been dramatically demonstrated in sensory-deprivation experiments in which the subject is cut off from practically all sources of stimulation, including other people. Unfortunately, this happens to a certain extent in many nursing homes for the elderly, where except for hurried and perfunctory attention to vital needs, the inmates are otherwise deprived of meaningful human contact and, in particular, of loving care. So they vegetate, deteriorating psychologically *and* physically. Those who have had a period of confined isolation from the outside world know how upsetting that can be. Being shut in for a while can make us actually yearn for the outside, crowded, noisy, or dirty though it may be at times. Absence of other human beings is especially painful, and we can become terribly lonely, depressed, and ill.

However, just as isolation can make us miserable, certain environmental stresses in the form of challenges—interesting problems at work, a complicated community issue, learning to ski—can be intellectually, emotionally, or physically rewarding. Stress, to some extent, is a necessary part of life, and in this form is *not* an indicator of impending illness.

EVERYDAY TENSIONS

But there are many stresses which tax our mind and body, and we vary in what and how much pressure each of us can take. What is shrugged off with little discomfort by one person becomes irritation, or even a forecast of sickness in another. Whether it's waiting to board a plane, being part of rushing humanity in heavy city traffic or crushing humanity in a department-store sale, sitting in the dentist's waiting room, standing in line to get a coveted seat to some sports spectacular, such everyday events start up the body's stress machinery.

And it is important to our health to be aware of, and to understand as much as possible, any such situations we really don't enjoy. If you find a department-store sale a nerve-wracking experience which leaves you with a big headache, it's a clue that you can't take it. A first step is to shop at a quieter time; giving your emotions and body an unnecessary beating isn't worth the money you save. (People for whom every penny counts may consider this suggestion a luxury, but actually it may help to avoid medical bills.)

If you find that your stomach knots and your hands get clammy when you ave to take a plane, or you get nauseated while riding in a car or train, then you might do your body a big favor by discussing this with your doctor so that he can throw some light on your anxiety (which usually is at the root of the symptoms) or at least prescribe some calming medication. These reactions are indicators that your body is, and could continue to be, a basic channel for discharge of tensions. Such everyday stress as a minor difference of opinion with a boss or a friend, annoying chores, an irritating social obligation, or a disappointing golf score, generally has only a temporary and small effect on us emotionally and bodily. If we find ourselves tense but with our bodies reflecting most of this in the form of indigestion, headache, constipation or diarrhea, backache, etc., and it's happening in lots of minor, everyday situations, that is a *message* that those situations are stressful for us and that we need to unwind. Why? Their cumulative effect might get close to what we would suffer over one major blow—such as losing our job. It is hoped that we will be motivated to consult our doctors or other health professionals, so we can be advised what steps can be taken to prevent repetition of the strain and worsening of our bodily discomfort.

STRESS IN DISGUISE

Another important thing to keep in mind is that when we undergo what on the surface appears to be insignificant stress, it actually may have a *hidden but important* meaning for us; thus some seemingly minor event can throw our whole body out of kilter and become an indicator of illness.

Recognizing your own private form of stress is easiest when it occurs in a dramatic and unambiguous fashion—a beloved relative suddenly dies, your firm goes bankrupt, your car hits a child. Such events will have a shocking effect—but in different ways for different people. You may be terribly upset right away or shortly after the experience has taken place, but you, and everyone else around you, expect such an emotional upheaval. What you may not know is that if you have shown little or no feeling at the time of their occurrence, such stressful events may trigger a later *physical* illness in you and therefore they are signs that should alert you to this possibility for a while afterward. It may even seem a mark of childishness or helplessness to become physically ill after an emotional upset, so we save our pride by attributing the illness to germs or some other acceptable alibi. Yet a dramatic shock is the easiest emotional indicator of possible physical disturbances to spot and then try to do something about. It's one of the few times when you can say to your doctor, "Look, I've just had a terrible thing happen to me—I want you to check me over." Your doctor's knowledge that you are under severe strain, and your own willingness to admit it, can help you both keep tabs not only on your emotions but also on your body.

Much harder to recognize as signals are those stresses that are not dramatic—the ones that are disguised to such an extent that we can easily overlook them. For instance, birthdays or anniversaries of deaths, weddings, graduations, promotions, the date we left home or our children left—these often have a hidden, *symbolic* meaning which can be very elusive and yet have the potential to affect our bodies. They may signify loss, disappointment, frustration, anger, the taking on of burdens, the beginning of many troubles. The more you're aware of these possibilities, the earlier you will be alerted to take measures to prevent severe mental *or* physical complications, especially if you find yourself not feeling up to par at the time of the anniversary.

Worry and guilt over sex are frequent causes of tension—whether you're just thinking about some forbidden erotic act, masturbating, or actually having relations with another person. If you experience these *feelings*, you'll tend to associate them with the sexual episode. But if, instead, they quickly fade into the background and you have a reaction in your *body* after the erotic activity, you'll probably chalk your discomfort up to something else. However, the rapid disappearance of tension and remorse are common signals that body disorders will follow sexual fantasies or acts. Often, after masturbation, you may suffer stomach cramps or diarrhea, neuralgic pains in the legs, frequency of urination. Your voyeurism may be followed by aching eyes or severe headache. After cunnilingus or fellatio you may be bothered by a sour taste in the mouth, trouble with your teeth, difficulty in swallowing, sore throat, nausea, or vomiting. Unsatisfactory sexual intercourse can give you strange or painful abdominal feelings, painful urination, or low back pain.

One of the most intriguing facts about our bodies is that we don't actually have to experience stress to have it physically reflected in us. Just *thinking* about something that might tempt us, seduce us, anger us, shame us, or *thinking* how we might win or lose a decision can be stressful enough to produce a physical reaction. So anticipating stress in our thoughts is a sign that our bodies may react. Suppose you had to give a little talk to your PTA and you didn't feel confident about how it would go over. Repeatedly you'd visualize the scene and get clutched in the pit of your stomach. When you'd eat you'd have indigestion. This would continue and even escalate right up to the time the talk was scheduled. If you had had colitis, a stomach ulcer, or other such ills in the past, they might be activated under these circumstances. The physical symptoms would be at their worst just before you spoke. Sometimes just acknowledging and reflecting on such (anticipatory) tensions can help put them in better perspective and possibly reduce them. Sometimes talking the situation over with another person, someone who is calm and reassuring, might help. However, repeated stage fright, actual or anticipated, really requires specialized attention.

In addition to stresses we overlook because they seem too insignificant to command our full attention, there are those we deny because they occur at times when we think we should *not* be under tension. In this category would fall the stresses we encounter on vacation, which will be discussed in detail in a later chapter. At this time, however, consider the popular belief that all persons—be they president, athletic celebrity, or private citizen—who engage in any sport for recreational purposes can only be enjoying themselves. At times that's true—but not always. Sometimes, say on the golf links, you simply can't escape from the pressures of work or marital difficulties, from other troubles and inner strain. You may still be fuming, full of guilt or apprehension, though it's not obvious to others—or even acknowledged by you. The presence of such tensions, the additional pressures of competitive anxiety, or too great a need to get a specially good golf score (and so feel you've succeeded at something!) may be enough to tip a *precarious though silent* balance between health and disease in the direction of sudden physical collapse. Disregarding these psychological warning signals can be risky. People who already have had a previous illness, such as a heart attack, from which they have recovered, may become especially vulnerable under such circumstances.

THE BLOOD CLOT OF SUCCESS

It may be difficult to believe, but success, as well as failure, can be stressful at times and can actually be a signal of impending illness. Here is an illustration. Wynn, at fifty, had only one rival for the top executive position in his firm after years of dogged work. His family had been urging him to let up, but he couldn't. Work helped him forget his guilt feelings. Many years before, he had been intensely jealous of his older brother, a talented violinist, who hogged all the parental attention while Wynn was neglected. Over and over Wynn had wished his brother dead. Then his brother, at the threshold of fame, developed polio and became a respirator case, a chronic invalid, paralyzed, unable ever to play again. Despite all the money he kept contributing to his brother's care, Wynn was like a haunted man—his hateful thought had come true, his brother was as good as dead. And so he worked to forget. When he got home he could hardly stay awake during dinner, but his sleep was troubled. In fact, he had been accumulating a sleep deficit for years. Weekends were for homework. Even the flu could not stop him from getting to the office. Vacations were horrible—he couldn't relax. Alcohol and sleeping pills made him feel worse.

It seemed like history repeating itself when his rival for the top position was suddenly felled by a stroke and Wynn had the job. That night he was enveloped by the warm glow of success—for the first time in many years he had a feeling of utter relaxation. It lasted only a few days, and then Wynn became obsessed with unrealistic thoughts that he had the job by default and had become number one just as he had when his brother was struck down. To counteract the severe guilt which had been stirred up, he immersed himself in work to prove himself worthy of the promotion. His sleep became more disturbed than ever. He had nightmares in which he stood astride the prostrate body of a man who looked like his former boss. During the day he found himself preoccupied with recollections of the trouble he had had with his brother when they were younger. Word filtered back that his rival was making an unexpectedly quick recovery. Wynn worked all the harder—again so he would have no chance to think about his hangups or feel any emotion. But this time he couldn't escape them. One night about a month later, he woke from sleep with terrible pain in his right leg. A blood clot had blocked a major artery there and he had to be hospitalized.

In neither instance was Wynn to blame for the tragic fate that overtook his rivals, yet because he had covertly wished them both out of his way he developed a hidden sense of guilt for what had happened to them. Success brings no happiness to people like Wynn; it only increases their suffering. If you have an overly strict conscience and go through an experience which makes you feel unnecessarily at fault, you may act to punish yourself in order to try to get some relief from your conscience. You might do this by working too hard and being overly concerned about whether you are doing a good job. But sometimes that combination isn't enough to neutralize stirred-up guilt. So a further increase in an already frenetic overactivity is attempted, and it bodes ill for you. It is a signal you're becoming vulnerable to a breakdown. These factors were operating in Wynn. They were warnings his health would suffer—and that's what happened. If you find yourself under such a terrible strain, simple awareness of your feelings will usually not be enough to help you resolve them and prevent their ill effect. Talking things over with your spouse or getting tranquilizers from your doctor may not be enough either. Psychotherapy then should be tried. It may enable you to understand how your emotions are doing you in and how you can best deal with them.

WHAT COMES AFTER LOSS?

In recent years a particular form of stress has been much studied. It is the actual, threatened, or symbolic loss of somebody or something emotionally significant to us. If we suffer a loss, and if no adequate substitute can be found, if our ability to adapt to loss is insufficient, if feelings of helplessness and hopelessness develop, then it is a sign our health can be profoundly affected. How long a loss affects us varies widely—for a day or two up to a year or more—though there are no fixed limits. Loss is not the *cause* of disease, but a common setting in which disease can develop.

If someone you love dies, you should watch your health and consult your doctor if you are at all under the weather, but especially if you feel helpless and despairing. Experiencing loss does not mean, however, that you *will* become ill. As I have already indicated, disease is not due to any one cause, nor is it signaled by any one thing—loss or anything else.

If you already have a chronic illness, loss may trigger a relapse, but the connection often is not apparent and not taken into consideration in the treatment. Here's an example in which I was able to help. At a hospital where I was a consultant, I went along with the professor of medicine to see a middle-aged woman who was in considerable distress. She had come in some days before because of a worsening, chronic heart condition. All the right things were being done medically, but she wasn't improving. We discussed whether psychological factors might be involved, but the resident in charge said quite emphatically that in going over details of the patient's personal life, he could find no evidence of emotional disturbance. On the contrary, she had told him how happy she was that she had just married off her last daughter a few weeks before.

Despite this, I was not convinced—sometimes people will *say* they're happy because they think they *should* be, when quite the opposite is true. Besides, aggravation of a chronic physical illness is *always* preceded by some emotional upset, even though that may not be apparent. So we decided to talk with the patient again. Yes, her daughter had just been married. To a wonderful young man. And they had gone off to live in Florida—so far away. This daughter had been her favorite, the last child, and now there were no more children at home. They had all grown up, married happily, and left her—suddenly the patient burst into tears and sobbed uncontrollably. Her brave front had broken down. She was really in mourning for her daughter, and for the years past when she had spent so much of herself on the children. And now all were gone.

She was happy for her daughter—in fact had tried not to deny any of her children happiness. But for the patient, who had neglected other interests and ways of finding pleasure in life, it had been a severe loss. Not wanting to admit this, she had been unable to adapt herself to it successfully. Her severe grief and confusion were reflected in her illness. She needed, in addition to her medicines, other treatment that would enable her to let out her true feelings, provide emotional support, and allow her to see the many options still open to her in this new phase of her life.

Thus separation and estrangement from someone close to us are warnings that our physical well-being may be affected. Yet the loss of another person is only the beginning of a long list of bereavements we can suffer. The loss of a pet may be keenly felt. If we lose a part of our body through injury or surgery, we also grieve. Giving up familiar surroundings at home and at work, or loss of prestige, reputation, money, or other external objects or symbols serving to maintain self-esteem, can make our emotions run the gamut from slight upset to real agony. Having to abstain from alcohol or some drug on which you have become dependent can cause distress. Even the discontinuance of an obsessive hobby can contribute to the sense of loss. Each loss should alert us to the possibility we may be physically vulnerable for some time afterward. Such danger will subside if we find adequate replacements for our losses.

RETIREMENT CAN PRESAGE ILL HEALTH

Retirement is one major change in our lives which—unlike some losses that come unexpectedly—we usually can do something about *in advance*. With proper planning and the right frame of mind, it can be a joy, a time to do things we never had time for before. But what occurs if we refuse or are just unable to think about retirement, pretending it won't happen? What if we then disregard any psychological (or physical) signs that our health can be endangered by the major change in our lives?

For forty years Ridgelow had run the laboratory in his own way. He knew he had reached the mandatory retirement age, but he couldn't believe it when the university authorities asked him to step down. The laboratory was his life. He spent practically all his working time in it or thinking about it, and he was not interested in leisure, or travel, or other forms of retirement. Ridgelow's social life was a blank. His wife had died twenty years before and there had been no children. Winding things down in the laboratory became increasingly painful as the deadline approached. Ridgelow began to think that perhaps he could find another place in which to continue his experiments. But he could find none. Outwardly he remained calm, optimistic, but inwardly the tension grew. What was he going to do? To cope with the loss of familiar instruments and co-workers seemed an impossible burden. Bitterness and anger welled up in him. How could they take away his laboratory? He was so upset that he even thought of burning the laboratory down. But he hid his rage, and finally he was unable to admit it even to himself. Time pressed him as he tried to pretend that leaving the lab just wasn't going to happen.

But then that day did come and he was out. To him it seemed he was out in the cold. He didn't know what to do with himself—even when he finally found a part-time job as consultant. His heart wasn't in it. He tried to stop thinking about his troubles and denied his feelings. Although he seemed to be calm, his tensions didn't go away. After several weeks in his new position, as he was leaving for home, he had a funny feeling in his chest. He didn't pay any attention to it and after a while it went away, but he was unaccountably tired. Following a couple of days of not feeling right, he went to see his physician. An electrocardiogram showed he had had a mild coronary thrombosis.

SIGNALS FROM THE ECONOMY

Statistics show that after economic recessions and depressions, there are increases in the number of heart attacks, ulcers, asthmatic crises, strokes, and other bodily ailments, as well as an upturn in mental hospital admissions. If you're a person who's apt to get physically sick under strain or who has had a chronic illness, these are times to be wary about your health. This is true particularly if you're suddenly out of a job with no prospect of getting another after being employed for years, if you've been unable to find employment over a long period of time, or if you're highly skilled and have to settle for a menial job.

On the other hand, employment does not guarantee emotional tranquillity or good physical health. If you can't adapt to stress easily, strained relations with co-workers and bosses at all levels of the organization will have some effect on you. So too will jealousies, rivalries, hatreds, back-stabbing, jockeying for favors. These are just as much an occupational hazard as a dangerous chemical, and continued exposure to them is a cue that your health may suffer.

SIGNALS FROM SCHOOL

Many children are exposed to fierce classroom competition and rising educational standards. If they are locked into such a situation by parents with neurotic ambitions, such children often will show signs of distress in the form of restlessness, irritability, poor appetite, fitful sleep, and repeated minor physical upsets. If the pressures continue unabated in children so affected, that's a signal that more serious trouble is likely—*physical* as well as mental. The breakdown may occur even in grade school. If it's in the form of behavioral disorder such as truancy, getting hooked on drugs, dropping out, flights into hippie culture and communes, or in the form of depression, psychotic episodes, or phobic reactions, it will be more readily correlated with stress. But the apathetic or seemingly compliant, goody-goody child often signals by these attitudes that the trouble is going to be in the body: colitis, asthma, migraine, skin disorders, menstrual difficulties, and many other disturbances. If the warnings go unrecognized, there's little chance that any preventive measures will be taken, especially to lessen the child's tension. Even after physical illness has developed in these youngsters, few doctors investigate the emotional factors.

SIGNALS FROM THE GHETTO

It is not only the ravages of malnutrition, unsanitary surroundings, drugs, and physical peril but, also the existence of terrible tensions which warn that the health of those who dwell in the ghetto is subject to danger. These tensions come from feelings of inferiority, frustration, hatred, and most of all from uncertainty about the future.

Paradoxically and tragically, ghettos may become the familiar and customary surroundings for the inhabitants —"their place." Many urban poor are uncomfortable outside their neighborhood. Sometimes, areas as little as a dozen or so blocks away are foreign territory. For some individuals, the immediate ghetto is a place where they feel they belong. Even if it is crowded, ugly, and shabby, it provides a kind of emotional security. Wretched as slum dwellings may be, they have come to represent the familiar; and with no other place available, they become emotional havens for many. Thus when slum dwellers are informed they have to move because their tenements are going to be torn down, and an uncertain future, especially in terms of a shelter, stretches before them, they are both furious and grief-stricken. Mourning occurs, comparable to that experienced when a loved one dies. Such a loss of "home" is stressful in the extreme, and is an indicator again that not only the psychological *but also* the physical life of the ghetto dweller can be affected most unfavorably, especially in the absence of adequate substitute sources of emotional support. Of course, the adaptive capacity of each person to such or any stress varies, and not everyone becomes ill. But a change from a place that is familiar and which you consider home, no matter how undesirable it may be, is another crisis in your life, another time when you must be on the lookout for unfavorable reactions in your body.

SIGNALS FROM UNUSUAL STRESS

What about war and combat? What do they do to the body as well as the mind? Young men—and in some instances young women—involved in the fighting are away from familiar surroundings and loved ones. They have been indoctrinated in the ways of destruction and death. The dangers that surround them are many and real. If they escape bombs and bullets, will illness be their fate anyway? Much has been written about the incidence of psychosis and psychoneurosis among military personnel, attributing these disturbances to psychological factors. But are there psychological signs that also forecast susceptibility to physical disease? Yes. These include stress from combat, previous bodily disorders when under strain, poor morale, attempted denial of emotional reactions to killing, sudden cessation of guilt feelings, dreams of bodily disturbance, persisting homesickness, and special preoccupation with thoughts about ill or dead relatives and buddies. The physical casualties predictable from those stress situations far outnumber those from enemy firepower.

Civilian populations are often directly affected by the ravages of war—by bombing, napalming, destruction of homes, starvation, and separation from loved ones. Extraordinary tension also prevails in urban and rural areas where religious, social, and nationalistic differences have led to continuing armed conflict, physical violence, and mass arrests. The common denominator in all such stress, and reinforcing it, is uncertainty. What dreadful thing will next happen to the individual, the family, the community? This question has been painted on walls and fences in various forms, most expressively as "Is there a life *before* death?" Again the focus has been on the mental breakdowns which occur under such dreadful conditions. However, disturbed emotions can also be early indicators of physical illness, particularly in the presence of inadequate food supplies, poor sanitation, and increased exposure to virulent germs.

INTERNAL CONFLICTS

Many have never experienced the horror of war or the degradation of the ghetto. Very few have been exposed to the extraordinary environments of the Antarctic, the space capsule, or most recently, the moon. But who, no matter in what society, has not experienced the usual vicissitudes of life, many of them man-made, related to human drives, needs, customs, and institutions? Who has not felt lonely and confined at times? Just as lack of food and water is harmful, so unsatisfied hunger for human contact hurts us. Many, many of us are isolated from others because of sexual inhibitions, competitiveness, timidity, fears, suspiciousness, and hatred—which may be reinforced by the kind of society we live in. We are driven by our emotions, restricted by our consciences, and subject to loneliness—the great predator. We are familiar with loneliness as a predecessor of emotional disturbances; however, it is also a prime sign of vulnerability to physical breakdown.

So all of us have to contend with *internal* stress, arising from biological processes in our bodies, activated by external events, and represented particularly by our sexual and aggressive drives—which relentlessly seek gratification. As these powerful forces push toward discharge in their own way, our consciences try to control their unbridled expression by psychological defense mechanisms. These defense mechanisms may not work; this is a sign that our bodies will take the full impact of these energies. So activated drives, insufficient defenses, and guilt which suddenly goes underground, are often predictors of impending physical disorder. From birth on, we try to deal with these internal pressures as well as with the stresses from the outside. Our childhood feelings which are closely related to these biological drives always attach themselves to the people who rear us. And the influence of these parental figures does much to shape our ways of coping with our sexual and aggressive impulses, and determines the formation of our conscience. Our struggle with our biological drives and our conscience, and the vicissitudes of our object relationships continue on through puberty, adolescence, adulthood, and the later years, though fluctuating in intensity and varying in form. Partly we're aware, partly we're unaware, of our efforts to deal with these inner conflicts. In turn, these *inner* psychological factors have a great deal to do with how we relate to other people and adapt to the outside world later. Yet they are often neglected as sources of stress and particularly as warnings of physical disease.

Stress always precedes disease, but does not necessarily lead to it. It is thus an important but *not* absolute sign that illness is in the offing. Stress may be followed by either emotional *or* physical illness; or by a state of dis-ease rather than any clearly definable sickness; or by little, if any, perceptible emotional or physical disturbance at all. Stress comes from internal conflict as well as from the external environment. However, we should also consider that stress will have a different effect on each of us because we are differently programmed by heredity in terms of our *potential* for health and illness. Our genes have some influence on when and how we get sick, as we shall see in the next chapter. We are also differently programmed, psychologically in particular, by our early experiences and development. In addition, if favorable life circumstances or relationships should follow our exposure to stress, they may have sufficient impact to neutralize it or compensate for it. That's when life itself is the psychotherapist, and when its influence may avert any illness or reverse its development.

Learning to be on the alert for stress is not always easy. Most of us have had the experience of thinking we knew someone very well, someone who seemed calm and unruffled, and then were surprised to find this person actually had been under great strain. This is not unusual, because generally we cover up our feelings. The façade we present —even to those closest to us—often doesn't reflect our inner tensions. This is true of us all. Even those of us who seemingly carry our hearts on our sleeves have secrets.

4

Like Parent, Like Child?

MORE THAN ONE POSSIBILITY

It seems as if some people are born destined to illness and others not. Some people become ill no matter how much they are spared from life's trouble. Others do not get sick even when they are subjected to great stress. Is heredity responsible? It's tempting to say that the kind of illness you'll get or the organ systems involved can be predicted from a careful examination of your hereditary background. Close to fifteen hundred human diseases are not considered to be genetically determined, though many are rare. But using hereditary data to forecast illness is not so simple. Often some aspects of an individual's heredity remain unknown or are inaccurate. In any event, such data are not specific enough. Other predictors besides heredity have to be taken into consideration. I refer particularly to psychological clues. These not only help indicate the most likely side of illness, but also the time of onset.

Each of us is born with a set of genes—the units of heredity which are complicated biochemical mechanisms. However, at any given time, parts of our genetic endowment, including susceptibility to particular illnesses, become very active or very inactive, depending on how we are affected by our internal and external environments. In any specialized body cell—for example, a nerve cell—only one-tenth or so of the genes in it (which influence its potential ways of functioning) are active at a particular time. Hormones and other substances *inside* our bodies can selectively suppress or stimulate this activity. *External* factors—whether they be exposure to viruses or an anger-provoking contact with someone—also can inhibit or activate our genes. But it is our involvement with other human beings—a most complicated experiential factor—which is so often overlooked as an indicator of how heredity and environment will interact to determine the state of our health.

Besides genes, other constitutional factors exert an influence after conception. For example, what happens within the womb plays a role in the embryo's development. If several embryos are present, their relative position, blood supply, etc., will influence their intrauterine development. But usually overlooked are the mother's anxiety or rage or her negative attitudes to the unborn child, her husband, and other members of the family—in fact, any emotional disturbance—which may upset her general physical health and, in turn, the normal physiology of her pregnancy. Nutritional supplies to the embryo, uterine contractions, hormonal balances, etc., are then affected. Conditions at the time of delivery, the interventions (such as anesthesia or forceps) required, and again, the mother's emotional state, will also affect the newborn.

PSYCHOLOGICAL CLUES, TWINS, AND DISEASE

The following case illustrates some aspects of the interaction between constitutional and environmental factors. But more specifically it shows how the mother's attitudes before birth provide clues to how she will react afterward and how this may affect the infant. Mrs. Duovem, in her mid-twenties, pregnant for the first time, was told by her obstetrician she would have twins. At first, she couldn't believe it. How would she find the time to take care of *two* babies, to love them, and also give enough attention to her husband? Gradually, helped by him, she tried to see the fun side of it. The disbelief, the anguish, seemed to fade away.

As she awaited the delivery, Mrs. Duovem became preoccupied with thoughts about the two in her. She felt that the one lowest down, the one who would come first, was the larger and kicked the most. The other seemed much smaller and quieter. She also assigned personalities to them. She thought the first one would be an active, restless type, getting into everything, whereas the second would be slow, steady, and deliberate. Mrs. Duovem was the youngest of a large family and had always felt she had been shortchanged in the attention and affection she got when she herself was a child. So her sympathies had always been with the underdog—the one getting the bad breaks.

Mrs. Duovem shared her speculations about the twins with her husband, who listened indulgently or seemed to. But his calm exterior was deceptive. Somewhat vaguely he sensed he wouldn't be getting all the attention he had become so used to during the first two years of their marriage. He even wondered if his old ulcer would flare up.

The first twin, a six-pound boy, was an easy delivery. The second boy, an identical twin, was a difficult business. He had to be maneuvered and extracted, and weighed in at under five pounds. Both babies cried vigorously and appeared healthy. Strangely, the parents had a name ready for the first one—Daniel—but hadn't yet selected a name for the second baby. In hurried and embarrassed consultation they finally agreed on Tod—for the husband's father, whose lingering death from stomach cancer had come just after their wedding. But who was thinking about *that*?

From the first day on, Mrs. Duovem saw Daniel as more substantial, needing her less than Tod, who, she thought, looked like such a sad little tyke. Tod had to go into the incubator, so he was left behind at the hospital for a few days. When he was finally brought home, he had become established as the weak one of the twins in the minds of both parents. He attracted more of the mother's attention, pity, and anxiety. She hovered over him and was uneasy when feeding him, and he responded by regurgitating his food and gaining little weight. He wanted to be held constantly. The big twin, Daniel, seemed to thrive and presented no problems at all. Two months later Tod had to be taken to the hospital for an operation. He had a condition called pyloric stenosis—a narrowing of the passageway from the stomach to the small intestine—which was successfully corrected by surgery. Hereditary factors pointing to the stomach as a vulnerable organ were so heavily represented in this family tree that it's not surprising to find the stomach was the site of physical difficulty. But Tod had also been handled with great anxiety by the mother. Was this relationship between infant and mother a precipitating factor in activating the condition toward which he was predisposed? Yes. The timing of the onset of his illness was not fortuitous but followed several months of this anxious interaction, which was a clue that the hereditary tendency might be activated. Afterward both parents tried hard to lessen Tod's burdens but unfortunately continued to be overly protective toward him. Whether Daniel, like his grandfather, his father, and his twin, would ever develop stomach trouble can best be answered by the following.

In twins, even identical twins, there are many other factors besides the particular kinds of genes each is born with which determine whether illness will occur—and what kind. But heredity *does* exert an influence. How much? Opinion varies. A recent study indicated that if an identical twin has an ulcer, the chances are one in four that his brother will have one too. (In fraternal twins there is only a one-in-ten chance that the other will develop an ulcer.) Though this indicates hereditary influence, it is important to keep in mind that 75 percent of identical twins and 90 percent of fraternal twins do not get ulcers. Therefore, *other* factors, that is, environmental ones, especially those concerned with the emotions, are involved in the development of ulcers. And how Daniel fared psychologically would be an indicator of whether his stomach would suffer.

We know that genes affect not only how our organs function, but also the chemistry of our bodies and the way we look. They are responsible for certain birth defects and inborn errors of development that may not show up until late in life and then only under special circumstances, among which the psychological are particularly important. Exposure to severe stress may set in motion a chain reaction of complex psychological responses which, in turn, become important signals that a hidden or latent potential for genetically caused disease is about to be activated.

HEREDITY AND ENVIRONMENT

In the case cited and in all instances of illness, is it heredity *or* environment? That's the wrong way to put it. Heredity *and* environment? Yes. But we don't know yet how much of each influences the development of physical illness. *That* remains to be determined by further research. We do know that our emotions are a prime source of signs pointing to the time *when* illness will occur. They may also add to our knowledge from other sources, medical genetics particularly, about where and what kind of disease is apt to develop.

Some years ago I saw in consultation a patient who presented a strong family history of breast cancer on the mother's side and arteriosclerotic disease (hardening of arteries) on the father's. She was an only child, in her thirties, much troubled about her hereditary background and the outlook for her health and longevity. Did she have cause for alarm? Well, many other factors need to be considered in addition to those derived from heredity. Without trying to list all of them, here are some of the more important physical ones: (1) Exposure to carcinogens, whether from radioactive substances, X rays, tobacco, or possibly certain viruses; (2) diet intake, heavily loaded with fat, cholesterol, or salt; (3) illness leading to residual organ damage, especially heart and lungs; (4) body trauma, acute or chronic, from injury or manipulation. But what are the signals that cancer or arteriosclerotic disease may be impending as a result of the confluence of these hereditary and environmental factors? In my opinion psychological clues will appear in many instances earlier than the physical ones, to indicate that an illness is developing. As we have already noted, exposure to stress, previous physical reactions to it, denial or general absence of emotion—anger in particular—sudden disappearance of remorse, blocking of psychological outlets, identification with sick or dead people close to us, and dreams of bodily sensation and disturbances should be looked for. Collating *all* these data would be representative of the interaction of heredity and environment and would provide more comprehensive information to patient and doctor about the possibility of disease and where in the body it may strike.

5

As Ye Adapt So Shall Ye Reap

LIFE STYLES

Our habitual ways of dealing with stress are also indicators of whether exposure to it will result in our becoming physically sick. Under ordinary circumstances, this *style of adaptation* fluctuates during our lifetime only within narrow, expectable limits. Some of us react by immediately becoming depressed when we face difficulties; others of us are characteristically more cheerful, tending to look for the bright side of things; still others develop physical symptoms. Thus, if we are aware that previously we have had trouble getting over disappointments or losses, then we have to be on the lookout for similar reactions whenever we face a current obstacle. Those of us who know we have adjusted to difficult periods in the past with relative ease may face new setbacks with some confidence. Thinking over past trials will help remind us whether our bodies were involved in these crises. Take, for example, the emotional setting in which we grew up. Did we, as children, feel very jealous of our siblings, constantly at odds with them and our parents, or did we think we were neglected, even unwanted? All kinds of reactions to these circumstances are possible. Some children show signs of emotional upset: They are cranky and anxious or they develop various phobias—especially about going to school; others are rebellious and accident-prone, or they exhibit behavior disorders; still others are sickly. Frequent colds, sore throats, stomach and bowel upsets, recurrent skin trouble, headaches, bedwetting, allergies, unusual susceptibility and severe reaction to the common contagious diseases of childhood, and a host of other physical disorders, indicate that reacting with the body may become the particular mode of adaptation to stress in childhood *and later in life.* Recollections from childhood may reveal that there were also "benefits" from being repeatedly ill—that it brought relief from stressful situations. For instance, Joey feels himself to be in the shadow of his brothers and sisters who he thinks are smarter, stronger, and more attractive than he. Furthermore, they are the focus of parental interest, and Joey feels neglected. This state of affairs is very troublesome to him. He can't cope with it psychologically. Then his body starts to act up. He can't hold food down and is terribly constipated. His weight drops. He is reacting to stress by developing a physical disorder. His sickness forces his parents to pay more attention to him. He has finally excelled in one thing—in sickness. This is a pattern which may repeat itself as Joey gets older, and may occur in other situations and in relation to other people. If this were something he or his doctor knew about, then prolonged physical illness following stress could be anticipated and, through proper therapeutic measures, prevented and averted.

Modes of adaptation to stress are, of course, never seen in pure form, i.e., just a physical *or* emotional response. They are mixtures of both. If you tend to react mostly with your body, there'll also usually be some psychological manifestations. For example, if your previous reaction when under a strain was to develop wheezing and difficulty in breathing—an asthmatic attack, accompanied by some feelings of sadness—then you can expect that exposure to a new, current, stressful situation will likely produce a recurrence of the more prominent physical condition, together with some emotional symptoms, probably depressive in nature. On the other hand, suppose previously you responded to stress by becoming so worried and upset that you couldn't do your work or enjoy yourself; and along with this you repeatedly got a cold or frequent headaches. Then you can anticipate that your response to future stress will probably be similar: a major emotional disturbance and a minor physical disorder.

ADAPTATION OUT OF KILTER

However, when stress is unusually severe or of a new and different kind, the mechanism of adaptation may go out of kilter, and then previous patterns of response aren't necessarily repeated. For example, assume your life has been free of major upsets and you now experience one of the following: loss of someone close to you, being uprooted suddenly from a familiar environment, financial disaster, unbearable marital troubles, or unpreparedness for retirement. Then you have to be on the lookout for changes in your adaptive response. Suppose, formerly, you released tensions by blaming others, having an angry outburst, or going off and acting impulsively. Now following the most recent stress, you react in none of these ways. You're apathetic, practically unable to do anything. That's a significant change in your style of adaptation, a sign that your body is bearing the brunt of the strain and that you soon may be coming down with a physical illness. Consider the following case: Tony, age thirty, had been an obsessional person for a long time. Whenever he was confronted with difficult situations, he became more rigid, more preoccupied with detail, less likely to have any feelings—in short, there would be an intensification of his obsessional traits. After he broke off with his girl friend, his only one since high school days, he tried to immerse himself in his work as an accountant—work which tended to be meticulous and exact. But he couldn't concentrate. He thought of going out with other girls, but didn't make a single date. He felt stymied, blocked, practically unable to do anything. After a few weeks, he developed a roaring case of colitis. This was the first time he had been physically ill and incapacitated since he was a youngster.

RETIREMENT BLUES

What happened to Ridgelow—whose case appeared in the previous chapter—is not unusual. We all know people who seem in good health as retirement approaches and who then suddenly become ill, or even die, when they have to give up their jobs. What clues in their mode of adaptation are useful in predicting this tragic outcome? Such people find it hard to give up the familiar, to become involved in new things and in a different kind of existence. They cannot easily step down from a position of authority or yield their niche, no matter how small, in the fabric of their working life. All this is suggestive of long-standing psychological rigidity. On retirement they are unable to cope with their aggressiveness which found a useful outlet in work. They cannot release it in any other way; they become immobilized, inert, and the aggressiveness is redirected against themselves, with disastrous consequences. When this happens and retired persons feel superfluous and finally useless, when their emotional dependency on others cannot be satisfied, these are warnings that they will become victims of early senility or some disabling disease of the body.

THE RIGHT SUBSTITUTE

We may all go through retirement, but some people have to face a different life earlier owing to divorce, widowhood, job obsolesence, etc. In fact, any significant change in a long-standing routine, a way of living, or a basic relationship with another person, will seriously tax our adaptive capacities, no matter what our age. Here again, we can look for a clue that will help us to anticipate what our physical health will be. This indicator is our ability to find adequate substitutes or alternatives for what we have lost or had to give up. Here's an example: Batch was a devoted son. In contrast to the other children, he visited his mother regularly, especially after she was widowed and lived alone. He saw to it that she did not lack money and kept a vigilant eye on her health, getting her the best of care. He didn't realize it, but some of his generosity was due to his never having quite freed himself from his mother's apron strings. There was a hidden, little-boy dependence left over in him. He got quite a kick out of his mother's praising him as a wonderful son—the only one of her children who was really attentive to her needs—even though occasionally Batch did feel burdened by his commitments and wished his brothers and sisters *would* share some of it. However, he pushed all negative feelings out of his awareness.

One day Batch's mother got a dizzy spell in the street and was struck by a car and instantly killed. When Batch heard the news, he was shocked. It was as if a big void had opened up in him. Though he'd been unaware of it, his visits with his mother had been major emotional experiences in his life, satisfying left-over needs for mothering. Over and over he recalled their many moments together, their long talks, the times she had been ill. A month after the tragic event, he continued to feel wrung out. He got a wicked cold which he neglected, and then one day he blacked out in his office. Alarmed, he finally went to his doctor for a checkup and was immediately hospitalized for a virus infection. For several weeks, Batch was very ill, more so than he had ever been. Even after he was released from the hospital he continued to have that empty, lonely feeling. He missed his mother more than ever. He didn't feel right, dragging himself around at work, still running a slight temperature. After several weeks of creeping convalescence he decided a vacation might do him good. On the cruise ship he met a widow, a bit older than he, who was warm, maternal almost, and very much interested in him. And then, for the first time in months, Batch felt less tense, less empty. His strength surged back and his temperature flattened out. He felt well again. Yes, he married the widow. Intuitively he had done the right thing—he had found a most adequate replacement for the great loss he had experienced. But many of us who are hit this way aren't so lucky. Our powers of adaptation or our circumstances don't lead us to the right solution or substitute for what we've lost. Life, which can be the great psychotherapist, passes us by.

ADJUSTMENT TO DISASTER

Hope—one measure of the self-preservative drives—often decides the struggle between life and death when the environmental stresses are extreme. Concentration camp victims—exposed to dirt, contagion, malnutrition, and brutality—who gave up hope died even if they did not go to the gas chamber. To be without hope is indicative of a profound breakdown in adaptive powers and is a basic sign that the physical health of prisoners in such grim surroundings will deteriorate rapidly.

Flood, earthquake, hurricane, and fire may destroy our material possessions and wreak havoc on our bodies as well as our minds. Even if we escape physical injury, the shock to our emotions may nevertheless make us vulnerable to some form of bodily illness. This is most likely to occur when disaster strikes suddenly and without warning. Suppose an earthquake leaves you homeless. You are physically unharmed; but what about your emotional reactions, particularly how you cope with catastrophe? If you feel overwhelmed, immobilized, helpless, and apathetic, this complex of responses is a sign that you are susceptible to *physical* as well as emotional illness. When a sense of loss begins to interfere with the initial feelings of relief at having escaped death, you may relive the disastrous event over and over. You may try to forget it. Or you may feel impelled to talk about it with anyone willing to listen. These are your attempts to adapt to the stress and the hurt it caused you.

Pre-existing difficulty in adapting and an ego easily shattered by severe stress will make recovery from the shock of the disaster complicated and slow. And not all the side effects will be psychological. Your body may be thrown off balance in various ways. Its resistance to infection, for instance, may be lowered just at the moment when faulty sanitation and crowded living in makeshift shelters drastically increase exposure to germs. An old heart condition may be aggravated. Arthritis that hasn't bothered you in a long time begins to kick up. So if your adaptation to stress in the past has been difficult and you become the victim of a natural disaster, this is a time to be especially alert to any unpleasant reaction in your body.

In less severe environments, adaptive capacity is also a basic predictor of whether illness will occur. Some of us find a way out by burying ourselves in work. Others become attached to a pet. Still others try ways of adapting that are just as amazing as those of the solitary prisoner whose coping ability is strained to keep his sanity and body from destruction. For him, improvising tasks with whatever objects are available, or becoming involved in the activity of any life which may be present—a bird, a mouse, even an insect —helps combat the harmful effects of isolation. A well-known example is the Birdman of Alcatraz.

People not in prison but unable to establish any real human relationships stave off psychological collapse by making radios their companions, to the extent that they are never without them. They carry their portables wherever they go, focusing on the sounds coming from them even as they walk among crowds of people. A few desperately use the telephone to get repeated weather reports and the correct time, just to hear a voice. These agonizing attempts to adapt are signs of vulnerability to further breakdown.

Most of us are not so badly off. Still we're not free of trouble, even though the strains are less severe and our adaptive capacities aren't so seriously taxed. In any event, it's useful to consider what your habitual mode of adapting to stress is. Do you get headaches, indigestion, the sniffles when you're under a strain? Or do you blow up, blame others, get depressed? Do you react mainly with your body or your emotions? That may foretell how you will react when you are confronted by more stressful situations. However, be prepared for the possibility that the familiar patterns of response may change, especially when you're exposed to unusual conditions. These are apt to so overburden your psychological coping mechanisms that other outlets for your tensions become necessary, and these outlets often take the form of serious bodily dysfunction.

6

Psychological Seesaw: Prelude to Physical Disorder

The tides of life fluctuate in us—but only within rather narrow limits despite great changes in our external environment; otherwise we would get sick or die. Such a relatively steady state is maintained in all our body functions and in our emotional reactions, while we're healthy. This is due to regulatory systems which control not only our metabolism, temperature, blood circulation, etc., but also how we think, feel, and behave in our interactions with other people.

DENIAL—USEFUL OR DANGEROUS?

When these balances are threatened, we get warning signals. The ones which are physical, such as rising fever, are well known, but those which are psychological have been overlooked. Here we will consider examples of the latter. The first is a process known as *denial*, which interferes with our perception of the world around us. It allows pleasant fantasy to be substituted for unpleasant reality and can be frequently observed in the remarks and actions of children. Studies of blind people indicate that this substitution occurs readily in them because they can't see certain disagreeable realities. It is also true for deaf people who cannot hear what otherwise might upset them. I know of two such people who had complications following an operation which restored

77

hearing. Thereafter, despite certain advantages from this change, they could not effectively deny certain aspects of reality which were very disturbing to them and which previously had been blocked off by the deafness. One became severely depressed. The other had a stroke. In adults a certain degree of denial serves two useful purposes: It prevents us from being distracted by trivia, and it also spares us unnecessary anxiety at times. But when we are exposed to continuous stress and depend on denial extensively to protect us from its harmful stimuli, that defense often won't work, and severe tensions will develop secretly in us. If these reach a critical point, we become mentally or physically ill.

Here is an example of how the tendency to deny unpleasantness immediately preceded awareness of a physical symptom in one of my patients. This occurred during a treatment hour. The patient had been talking at some length about his troubled marriage and appeared to be under considerable tension. In the midst of his discourse, the following thought intruded: "In spite of all the disagreements with my wife, I haven't had any headaches." That was the denial. A few minutes later he became aware of pain in the back of his head. For the rest of the hour he complained of a nagging headache. In this instance, denial was ineffective in blocking unpleasant physical sensations activated by recollections of his domestic difficulties. Actually, it signaled the breakthrough into consciousness of his body sensations.

Another patient, whom I saw in consultation, was a habitual denier. Whenever anything came up in his thinking or in conversations with others which was unpleasant or irritating, he would say, "Forget it. No use in thinking about it. What's done is done." His wife was that way, too. Having recently retired from his job as foreman in an industrial plant, and feeling at loose ends—without any plans for the future and insisting that he wasn't the least bit disturbed by this major change in his life—he caught a cold which didn't get better. He felt unusually tired, lost some weight, and looked pale. But he insisted it was "nothing," simply the virus which had hung on. His wife went along with him. Even when his gums began to bleed profusely, something that had never happened before, he ascribed it to eating too many soft foods. He insisted there was no need to have his condition checked out. So he denied and denied—and died of acute leukemia.

If you are a *habitual* denier and are developing a physical illness, you may not notice internal sensations of very low intensity from the affected bodily area for some time before actual symptoms break into your awareness. Even then the process of denial may make you belittle the significance of such symptoms or simply disregard them. In any event, by the time you get to a doctor, things may have progressed unpleasantly far. That doesn't necessarily mean that you will be found to have an incurable disease. However, if you are aware of your tendency to deny disagreeable reality, you often can prevent a prolonged siege of illness by getting the necessary medical attention early, when you first feel indisposed.

NO FEELINGS

When we have little awareness of our feelings, a condition called affect block, we may be spared discomfort from them, but at a price. We are cold, emotionally unresponsive, and do not relate well to other people. If we express feelings explosively but have no understanding of their meaning, we also may find ourselves in trouble. These emotional spurts which relieve our tension only briefly aren't worth the additional difficulties they create for us. But with either kind of response, a time will come when we are under great pressure and these defenses will not work; our equilibrium will be upset, and physical complications will develop. The intense energies associated with our feelings, if inadequately discharged or dealt with through our psychological systems, will have a disruptive impact on our bodies. So, if you are inclined to be an unfeeling person or one who blows up easily without really understanding why, and you find yourself in a very stressful situation, watch out! You may be on the way to developing a physical illness.

Donna, in her mid-thirties and doing well as an advertising agency executive, was secretly dissatisfied with her bachelor-girl status. You wouldn't have known it by her serene, cool, even aloof demeanor. She had come from a family where expression of feelings was discouraged and considered in poor taste. By concentrating on her work and on what made other people tick, she avoided thinking about her own personal problems. And so, for a long time she maintained this balance. When Donna unexpectedly lost one of her most important accounts, she seemed unperturbed. People at the agency were not surprised at her calm; after all, nothing ever fazed her. A week later she was stricken with pleurisy. She had shown no feelings under stress, but this time the equilibrium had not been maintained. Blocked from expression and more intense than ever before, her emotions had nowhere to go and struck with full fury at her body.

IDEA BEFORE SENSATION

Another sign indicating a shift from psychological to physical expression of tensions is finding yourself preoccupied with bodily sensations which previously were absent or fleeting. For instance, you become aware first of a *thought* about fullness in the front part of your throat. This intrudes unpleasantly into consciousness and increasingly distracts your attention from other things if you don't make any effort to shut it out of your mind. Later you become aware of the *sensation* of fullness. What can it be? A physical equivalent (representation) of anxiety or depression; or a hysterical conversion reaction (symbolic manifestation of an underlying sexual conflict); or a very early signal that your thyroid gland is not functioning properly. A physical checkup together with an evaluation of your emotional state will indicate which of the conditions it's likely to be.

I have noted many instances where the *idea* of the physical sensation comes into awareness *before* the physical sensation itself. So *that* becomes a very early signal that a body disturbance which may be minor or major is in the making. A number of my patients mentioned they were having thoughts that their heart beat was becoming irregular some minutes or longer before the extrasystoles (skipped beats) or auricular fibrillation (gross disturbance in rhythm) actually began. This was in the context usually of preoccupation with troublesome events or in anticipation of these. Other patients anticipated a bout of diarrhea (before they had experienced any physical warnings that it was going to occur) by having angry thoughts and feelings of exploding—again in relation to a situation of stress.

The persisting tendency to deny unpleasant thoughts and situations is an indication that sooner or later your body will become vulnerable to the impact of tensions which actually have not been released. If you're a person who cannot express your troubled feelings readily, such an interference is also an indicator that any secretly escalating strain can eventually make itself felt through gross bodily disturbances.

BLOCKED PSYCHOLOGICAL OUTLETS

But by far the more important indicator of vulnerability to physical illness is a shift in our emotional equilibrium which progressively blocks the discharge of our tensions through *all* psychological outlets, i.e., through the processes of thinking, feeling, and behavior. Bodily pathways are substituted for psychological pathways in an attempt to release the pent-up energies. It is then that the likelihood of our developing physical disorders, minor or serious, becomes very great. So, we look for evidence of low-keyed manifestations of tension after stress—evidence which otherwise might be casually dismissed because it is not in the form of any dramatic psychological symptoms. Examples include constriction of fantasy life, dullness of emotional response, and absence of "acting out" (neurotic behavior).

7

Rage: The Misunderstood Clue

While speculation on *how* hostility contributes to bodily disorders continues, its importance as a clue to predicting the development of illness has been overlooked by many doctors and is unknown to most people. Consider the following: Do you have reasons, because of jealousy, rivalry, criticism, disappointment, loss of emotional support—realistic or irrational—to be angry at other people but are unaware of this feeling? Or if the rage is at first out in the open, but then disappears, do you think of what happened to it? The key question is then: Where did the anger go? You'll find that it's often directed against yourself. In turn, that means either you'll get depressed or come down with a physical illness.

Consider this situation: You have broken up with someone close to you on whom you depended for advice, guidance, and reassurance, though you didn't always get it. Since then you have been unable to find any replacement for the relationship. What follows? Hostility toward your friend for leaving you builds up and seeks an outlet. If none is available, if the anger can't be adequately dissipated, that is a clue that the pent-up feelings will hit your body, which cannot handle this overload of energy. The result is a disruption of normal physiological and biochemical processes.

WHERE DID THE ANGER GO?

Your boss, who has been riding you for weeks, has just chewed you out again for a trivial mistake you made at work. You feel like killing him but control your anger, just as you did when as a child you were scolded by your father. Then, Mother had warned you not to upset him because it might make him sick. He suffered from what you later learned was an ulcer. Now after the scene at the office, when you return home, you slouch around, unusually silent. The next morning you're back at work but numb. You've pushed the whole ugly incident out of your mind. No feelings, no thoughts about it. When you had those run-ins with your father, you would have an upset stomach for days. But now, nothing—at least for a while. Then you begin to have a general feeling of malaise. But where's the anger? Some hours later, during a coffee break, you suddenly feel as if a lightning bolt had struck you in the solar plexus. When you're rushed to the hospital, every effort is focused on your physical condition. Did anyone, yourself included, stop to think that your bottled-up anger was a sign that you might get sick? And what might have happened if that signal had been picked up early? Anger could have been drained off then through less harmful means and your body might well have been spared.

UNFAMILIAR FORMS OF HOSTILITY

Often anger is difficult to detect because it has become locked up in an emotional conflict and is then expressed in disguised ways. Ruth worked for a state agency dealing with all aspects of racial discrimination. She was in charge of the typists, and under her direction the correspondence from the agency was done promptly and usually letter-perfect. Outside of work, Ruth was given to expressing herself rather freely about what she felt were undesirable traits in certain ethnic groups—their pushiness, arrogance, money-grabbing, etc. This never happened when she was on the job. Ruth suffered from severe migraine headaches and had talked over her disability with a psychologically perceptive consultant. From him she learned to her astonishment that she was a very angry woman. She hated lots of people and wasn't really aware of it. Ruth had fought off her own sense of inferiority by focusing on what she would call, all too readily and unreastically, defects in others because of their race and ethnic origin. And yet she had a job in the very agency that had been set up to combat discrimination.

Anger can be concealed by an opposite attitude. Some people are able to achieve this relatively stable psychological defense—called reaction formation—against their sadistic impulses. The defense may be effective for a long time, though there may be some "leakage" in the form of occasional symptoms such as irritability, headache, insomnia, etc. However, it is apt to collapse if stress from within or without becomes too great. Under these circumstances, the rage which has been internally bound by reaction formation is released. A new psychological outlet for it may become available. For example, the "nice person" will become an "angry person." If such release is not possible, and the "nice person" becomes a "depressed person," that is a sign the unbound anger is still turned inward, but wreaking havoc psychologically. However, if the "nice person" ends up by experiencing no feelings, that person's body will take the impact.

Hostility as a factor in physical illness has been known for many centuries. Its influence has been described in primitive, magical, religious, philosophical, and romantic terms. In recent years psychological explanations of its role in disease have become more sophisticated, though they're still incomplete. However, what is more useful for you is knowing as much as possible about the ways you deal with your anger. Then you'll be better able to understand it as an indicator of illness. In particular, absence of anger or its disappearance when it should be evident in our thoughts, feelings, or behavior suggests the likelihood of a breakdown in our physical health. It also predicts when an already established illness is apt to get worse. This is illustrated in the following case.

Lottie had had rheumatic heart disease since the age of thirteen, with occasional relapses requiring hospitalization. Her brilliance at school was followed by a rapidly successful career in a large corporate firm. Her advancement was furthered by her great ambition and drive to overcome her physical handicap. She had a beautiful sister who became a famous model. Both had grown up in a home where their mother, deserted early by her husband, had taken a job as housekeeper (and mistress) to a rich widower with children of his own. The mother had repeatedly warned her daughters to be seen and not heard, to be as unobtrusive as possible, and to avoid fights with the other children and between themselves. She did not want her position in that home to be jeopardized in any way.

Lottie, the nice, the brilliant, the successful, seethed with hatred but didn't know it. She hated her father whom she hadn't seen since childhood. She hated her mother and her mother's lover. She hated the other children who had all the advantages and her own sister who was more beautiful.

I first saw Lottie in consultation after she had married and found that she and her husband could not agree on anything—she, quietly and he, loudly. He had turned to other women. It was quickly apparent that originally her illness and the subsequent recurrences had been signaled by critical escalation of hostility which had no place to go except against her body. Episodes in which she felt, often inappropriately, that she was being humiliated or had to be very competitive or in which she experienced uncompensated dependency needs, all invariably triggered the anger.

And now it was the impasse between herself and her husband which threatened her wellbeing. I warned her that she urgently needed attention for her emotional problems and a chance to become more aware of her hostility in order to lessen it; otherwise her heart would again fail her.

She was in treatment with me for two years during which her relationship with her husband improved somewhat, and she had no relapse physically. We had made a solid start toward getting her anger out from under the repression which had buried it, and also we had begun to shift its impact away from her body. Then, suddenly, her husband left her. Her extreme anger showed briefly and then went underground. She seemed in emotional shock. Her need for psychotherapeutic help was greater than ever. But she left treatment and moved to another city where she made plans to undergo cardiac surgery. Some months later I learned she had died before any operation could be performed.

8

When a Bad Conscience Affects Health

THE MANY FACES OF REMORSE

Ordinarily, if we feel remorseful, we show it in a variety of ways. Many of these are psychological and are more or less hidden in what we're thinking, feeling, or doing. So our sense of guilt often is not easily recognized by us or by others. It may be experienced as dull tension, feelings of being slowed up, a reluctance to do anything, or a need to ingratiate ourselves with others. There also may be expectations of catastrophe, unusual feelings of humility, a need to be punished or purified. Sometimes we get into what seems an endless series of failures, of acts of expiation and renunciation. The need for punishment may so dominate a person that he commits a real crime in order to find some justification at last for his tormenting remorse and then get relief by being caught and punished. Occasionally, we take the sins of others upon ourselves, and this comes to represent a borrowed sense of guilt.

Suppose you have been flirting with a colleague's wife and have thought of having an affair with her. Usually you react by feeling uneasy every time you think of the possibility or whenever their names are brought up in conversation. Though you deny to yourself there's anything wrong, and explain your desires as mostly fantasy, you continue to feel strained. Or you may indicate indirectly by your behavior that you're troubled: You suddenly find that you've carelessly burned your hand, cut your finger, or twisted your ankle.

These are disguised ways in which we show guilt, or our need to hurt ourselves, through our behavior.

But what if we've been through a shocking experience which has stirred up much guilt, and then after a while we don't feel remorse or show *any* psychological manifestations of it. That is a prime sign that physical suffering is about to be substituted for emotional suffering.

I saw a patient several times in consultation who was troubled about the state of apathy he had fallen into after having been an active man for many years. He was a bachelor in his forties and had devoted his energies exclusively to ventures in the restaurant business. Now he was without a store, waiting for an opportunity to acquire one. But something was dampening his usual enthusiasm and drive.

He told me his father and mother both had been rigid and harsh. Discipline was their key word. For years, except for attendance at school, he was kept quite isolated at home. His parents, well-off and ambitious for him, insisted that he study all the time, even while other children were out having fun. Meals were eaten at an exact hour every day. He recalled how during dinner he could hear the shouts of children playing nearby, but didn't dare ask to be allowed to go out. He suffered a lot from indigestion. Instead of baseball or sledding he was expected to practice the violin. His parents tolerated no disagreement with their decisions and permitted no discussion. Otis hated them, and he grew up a seemingly compliant, but inwardly rebellious, child. Several times he dared run away from home, but he was quickly brought back by the police. Masturbation was his secret consolation when things seemed at their worst, and his fantasies were full of sadistic and masochistic sexual scenes.

Otis went through college a loner, and after finishing there he never returned home. He had become increasingly interested in food processing and was able to get several jobs in that industry. Some years later his parents died, one shortly after the other. He was unable to mourn their passing, but took the modest inheritance they left him and put part of it into a restaurant. Then followed an extraordinary pattern of success and failure. As long as he maintained one restaurant he did very well. As soon as he established the second he felt impelled, despite his know-how, to do all the wrong things. The result was bankruptcy. He wasn't down for long. Starting from scratch and using the rest of the inheritance, he developed another successful restaurant. And again when he started a second, he failed. The third time around, being without capital, he took a partner. Once more the business prospered, but this time when Otis wanted to add another restaurant, his partner disagreed. They quarreled violently, and finally Otis was forced to sell his share of the business.

While he waited for another opportunity which didn't come, he watched his former partner develop several other successful restaurants. Otis went through a dreadful few weeks, devaluing and denouncing himself for all his mistakes. He couldn't eat and his sleep was fitful, but worst of all he increasingly berated himself for everything—not only his business misjudgments, but his hatred of his parents, his indifference to their death, his squandering (as he now saw it) of the inheritance, his solitary life, his masturbation. It seemed as if he had done nothing right. And then suddenly the emotional storm seemed to be over. The remorse faded away, leaving him feeling dull and apathetic.

That is when Otis consulted me. His harsh conscience for years had been taking its toll by forcing him into neurotic actions which undid each venture of his that promised to be successful. Despite his periodic attempts to free himself from his tyrannical conscience, he was unable to. It was clear from his remarks that he was still searching for a way out of his dilemma, though he did not appear either angry or sad and seemed to have no guilt. This absence of feelings was an ominous sign of trouble still brewing. It suggested that the tensions between himself and his conscience had not abated but had only shifted the direction of their thrust, and now they would probably strike at his body. I advised him to get into therapy immediately to relieve the intense strain he was under. Otherwise he soon might become physically sick. He wanted a few days to think it over, but I next heard from him somewhat later, after he had been operated on for a bowel obstruction.

NOW YOU FEEL IT, NOW YOU DON'T

Extreme conditions, such as exist during war, may influence both conscience and body in extraordinary ways. This is demonstrated in a study of successful and highly competitive business and professional people suffering from ulcers who became prisoners in World War II. They were studied before, during, and after their imprisonment in a European concentration camp. An amazing shift occurred from physical illness to behavioral disorders while they were prisoners. During their exposure to extreme hardships and suffering, most of them were not troubled by ulcer symptoms; no longer did they have stomach pain and indigestion. Instead they experienced intense fear and hatred, lost their ambition, and abandoned their moral and ethical standards. They were openly greedy, irritable, and scheming, and were concerned only with themselves. After they were released from the concentration camp and returned to their former environment, they again developed symptoms of peptic ulcer and reverted to their old personality patterns. They again became prisoners of their consciences.

So ill health often has a symbolic significance: atonement for neurotic guilt. When our lives are threatened, and we are confronted with extreme danger and suffering, the remarkable shifts noted above can take place. Experiencing great physical discomfort and mental anguish appears to be atonement enough. We no longer need to be sick or hurt ourselves to do penance. Under these circumstances, our aggressive impulses are turned away from our bodies and against the outside world, against other people—even fellow sufferers.

There are times when remorse surfaces to consciousness only briefly or not at all, though you've been through a tough time. It remains hidden, without psychological manifestations such as overt depression, sad thoughts, or self-destructive behavior. That is when remorse becomes potentially deadly for your body, when your body will be a prime target for piled-up inner tensions and will be especially vulnerable to other disease-producing factors.

9

Dreams That Signal Sickness

ANCIENT BELIEFS

Even when illness is in its earliest stage of development and no symptoms or signs have yet appeared to warn you or alert your physician, you may actually learn of its presence through *dreams*. Man has always been fascinated by dreams, and his understanding of them has been closely related to the cultural stage of his development. For example, primitive people consider dreams to be the work of supernatural beings who reveal their evil intentions of sickness or death through this medium. Some primitives avoid waking a sleeper because they believe his soul is away during sleep and if he is awakened before the soul returns, he will fall sick or die.

For centuries people who were under the influence of theistic religions considered dreams to be divine communications. Consequently, for them dreams had a prophetic significance, especially in reference to their health and well-being. Many other people emphasized the physical basis of dreams, attributing either little or no meaning to them, or else they considered dreams to reflect some body disturbance. In ancient China dreams were thought to be warnings of impending illness when the Yin and Yang symbols (two polarities of a vital force) in them were found to be out of balance.

MODERN STUDIES

Modern studies indicate that changes in our bodies, which subsequently may be associated with disease, are first registered in our brains at a level below consciousness. So, at the very beginning of a potential illness we are not directly aware that anything is wrong when we are awake. And, if we are habitually deep sleepers, the physical sensations are not strong enough to disturb sleep. However, though the stimuli coming from the affected area are initially weak, they mingle in our minds with other stimuli from events in our daily life. If these impressions are associated with forbidden wishes and neurotic fears of punishment, they can stir up repressed memories of related experiences from our past. This combination influences dream formation. Consequently, hidden in the tangled web of our dreams may be the first hints of a body disorder as well as fulfillment of infantile expectations. What links them together is the common denominator of a wish—a wish for relief of tensions, discharge of accumulated stimuli, atonement, etc. However, should we be light sleepers and should these same body excitations increase somewhat in intensity, they will likely awaken us. We then may be briefly aware of them before we fall asleep again.

MARRIAGE ASKEW

Here are some illustrations: Jonny felt very tense after his fiancée pressured him into setting a wedding date. Though bright and well educated, his long-standing sense of insecurity prevented him from using these assets. He fumbled his way from one job to another and also from one girl to another, till this last one who held on to him. Actually he had never resolved his awe of his athletic father and brothers who frequently poked fun at him as the runt of the family. He remained terribly self-conscious about his size, though he was now an adult. Secretly he wondered whether he could face the responsibilities of marriage. Though no one knew it, he wished he could back out of his commitment. One night shortly before the wedding date, he dreamt that he was trying to make his way through a room filled with people at a party. In the dream he was powerfully built, especially about the neck and shoulders. By twisting and turning, but with much discomfort, he finally forced his way out of the crowd. His associations to the dream indicated that he was trying to turn away from the wedding, that the prospect of getting married terrified him. In addition, his long-hidden wish to be physically more powerful than his father and brothers was evident. At the same time his deep sense of guilt about these desires was also apparent. But the dream also was a sign that something was happening to Jonny's body, even though he had not experienced any physical symptoms as yet. Then, two days later, Jonny developed acute torticollis (wryneck) and had to wear a plaster of paris collar around his neck for weeks. The wedding date was postponed.

A DREAM OF GROWTH

One of my patients, Agatha—a graduate student—had entered treatment because of a serious work block. She was very bright, but because of her perfectionistic tendencies and excessive attention to detail she had been unable to finish her thesis. Though married for several years, she had deferred having children until she received her Ph.D. Her husband, an older man who taught in the same university, seemingly deferred to her every wish. Agatha was highly competitive, not only with other students, but with the professors, including her husband. She came from a small family, being the elder of two girls. Her father was athletic coach at the local high school and her mother was a teacher there. Both parents were obsessional, cold people. As a child Agatha felt her father didn't like her because she wasn't a boy. Her mother, always busy with school work, with "the other children," seemed to have little time for her. The younger sister had married early, after finishing high school, and was busy raising a big family. Agatha secretly envied her sister's apparent contentment. Her own marriage had cooled down after a brief romance, and Agatha and her husband had lost interest in each other physically.

The early part of treatment was marked by Agatha's attempts to prove she was the best, the most knowledgeable of my patients. But she showed little feeling; it was all expressed in words. Some months later she learned her husband was playing around with another woman. This elicited some anger. Then she was told to be ready for a general examination in the subject on which she was writing her thesis. This evoked anxiety. For the first time she mentioned a physical complaint—easy fatigability—although she had enjoyed good health for years. Then she had a painful menstrual period, which was an unusual occurrence for her. Shortly afterward I had to be away for a few days. On my return, it was clear that Agatha's anxiety and irritation were mounting. Her thoughts reflected her concern with the theme of what would happen to her at the hands of men. Her next period was late, and she referred to a feeling of fullness in her abdomen. Then she had a dream in which she was attached to a balloon which lifted her higher and higher into the air, when suddenly it burst, and she plummeted to earth. She awoke in a fright. Her associations indicated how much she wished to be free of all her troubles and yet felt that they would do her in. A few days later she dreamed she was swelling up, that everybody thought she was pregnant, and that she had to urinate urgently. Her associations revealed her envy of her sister's fertility and her own wishes and fears about having children. In the same hour she mentioned a new physical sensation: pressure on her bladder. She wondered if she indeed were pregnant. I considered that the dreams were indications of some hidden physical disorder and urged her to consult with her gynecologist (because other conditions than pregnancy also might be responsible for her symptoms). It turned out that she had an ovarian cyst.

PRECURSOR OF MENSTRUATION

Dreams of illness or dying do not necessarily portend such an outcome. For instance, one of my patients, a woman in her late thirties, had become upset because she feared she would not be able to have a baby. She had just married, but could not get pregnant. She and her husband had had an extended honeymoon. Later she told me about the following sequence of events. As the honeymoon neared its end she mentioned to her husband in casual conversation that she was premenstrual. Then she forgot about it. That evening they played Scrabble at which she was very good, winning both games. Before bedtime, her husband had a drink, while she munched on cheese and crackers, and she again remarked she was premenstrual. What she didn't tell him was a fleeting thought which had crossed her mind: She was getting along in years and she wondered if she would ever be a mother. That night she had a vivid dream, remembering when she awoke only that it had to do with painful dying. She felt quite anxious and wondered during the morning if she were going to be ill, perhaps seriously. That afternoon on the beach she forgot about her worries as she noticed how many admiring looks she got in her stunning bikini. When she and her husband finally got up to leave, a red splotch marked the white fabric. These events appeared first in her recollections when she resumed her interviews with me. The dream had heralded her menstruation, and she indeed had dyed (her bathing suit). The dream was another disguised indicator of her intense disappointment at not being able to become pregnant.

FORECAST: BACKACHE AND HEMORRHOIDS

Here is a different kind of dream, one which at first telling contained no hint of illness or disability. A male patient of mine, generally well except for occasional minor ailments, had taken a few days off from his job in an advertising agency after beating out a rival in getting a long sought after account. He went to a fancy mountain resort but resented having to lug his suitcase a short distance at the airport when no porter was available. He was an egotistical, exhibitionistic kind of person, as yet only beginning to be aware of how ingrained these traits were. That evening, entering the grand dining room of the hotel for dinner, he felt uneasily self-conscious. However, he became angry at the head waiter who seated him at a corner table, away from the glitter of all the beautiful people. So he didn't enjoy the elaborate meal. Afterward he felt tense. That night he dreamed of going to the premier preformance of a new play. In the dream he didn't like his seat and paid an usher to get him a better one. As a result he found himself with his back to the stage, facing the audience in a very uncomfortable position.

When he told me about it on his return, the associations pointed to his having been anxious about the fancy hotel, feeling out of place, then about being snubbed and relegated to an inferior place. He developed rage and guilt as a result, then "feeling nothing," he went to bed. All this suggested he would probably have some bodily repercussions. Indeed, the next afternoon he developed a severe spasm in his lower back. It gradually improved, but on the second day of vacation the patient became constipated, strained at stool, and developed an extremely painful hemorrhoid.

BODILY SENSATIONS IN DREAMS

While dreams are a source of very early signals that disease is developing, their significance in this respect is not often readily apparent. The manifest content of a dream can be deceptive. You may remember dreaming of illness and that may not have been the real meaning of the dream at all. On the other hand, a dream at first glance may contain no reference to disability or ill health. This may become apparent only after your associations to the dream are available for analysis. It is difficult for the lay person to analyze dreams or get at the significant associations to them. A competent professional's help is usually needed for this. However, the repetitive appearance of references to bodily sensations in dreams is suggestive of some hidden physical disorder. Dreams are infrequently the sole signals of developing illness. They are usually accompanied by other psychological predictors. Under such circumstances our dreaming may indicate the presence of bodily dysfunction which is as yet not manifested by distinct physical symptoms and signs or even detectable by the most modern laboratory tests.

10

When a Body Imitates a Body

SOMATIC IDENTIFICATION

The tendency to imitate others through physical response is a very common trick our minds play on us when we're overly preoccupied with our bodies. For instance, if you read about an appendectomy, or someone tells you about his, you may begin to feel twinges of pain in the right side of your abdomen, even if nothing is wrong with you. Medical students and nurses in training often think they have symptoms of diseases they are studying. While these are relatively simple examples, our minds can play similar tricks on us in more complicated ways. All of us tend to take on the characteristics of other people when our relationship with them assumes a certain emotional significance for us, for example, when we admire them and want to be like them; or when we lose them or are disappointed in them and need somehow to cling to them; or when we are afraid of them and try to avoid our fears by becoming like them.

This phenomenon, called identification, generally has been considered to be a process that follows psychological lines; for example, our ways of speaking, tone of voice, mannerisms, personality traits begin to resemble theirs. But identification also has strong physical roots. The term "somatic identification" refers to resemblances between ourselves and the person important to us which are manifested in posture, gait, and appearance, as well as symptoms and signs of illness, or illness itself.

TWO CASE REPORTS

Suppose a person very close to you, such as your brother, dies, so that you experience a terrible loss. You may not be able to get him out of your mind; an extraordinary concentration of your thoughts and feelings are on him. In the past the two of you were frequently at odds. As children you scrapped a lot, were treated differently by your parents, and were intensely competitive with each other. Now, however, you may take on not only the psychological but the *physical* characteristics of your brother, yet for the most part you are unaware that this is happening. You begin to talk or act like him, assume his posture, gait, and mannerisms. Or, without your knowing it, changes take place in your physical functioning until symptoms resembling his start to trouble you. Your brother's illness was due to cancer of the stomach. You were with him a great deal before he died. Your many impressions of how he looked, sounded, smelled, and acted are vivid ones, imprinted on your mind. Especially his inability to eat, his vomiting, his pain, his wasting away, his terror as death approached.

If you had been aware of this very close identification and of its significance indicating vulnerability to physical disorder, you would have at least been alerted to the possibility that, should you get sick yourself, it might be in the same bodily area. But some months after his death, the impressions of your brother have faded from your awareness, though you continue to miss him and have found adjustment to his absence a difficult one. Now you notice that your appetite is poor, that you're having a lot of indigestion, and that you've lost some weight. Your doctor says you've got gastritis (an inflammation of the stomach).

Here's another example. Len had developed a curious weakness of the right hand. He couldn't hold a pen or pencil in it, though otherwise it didn't bother him. Neurological examination at first revealed no positive findings. I was called into consultation. Talking with Len at some length, I learned his father, with whom he had always been rivalrous, had recently had a stroke which paralyzed his right side. Len had been very upset by this. It seemed as if his condition was an hysterical conversion response to the father's illness. But I had noted, behind Len's concern, signs of intense hostility to the father which was largely repressed. I also thought that there was increasing evidence that psychological outlets for his disturbed state were becoming insufficient, that his conflicts were being bottled up, and that the so-called conversion symptom in his right hand might not allow for adequate discharge of his emotions. I advised that he be given some immediate psychotherapy to release the tensions in him. He refused treatment.

Some time later, I learned that he had been readmitted to the hospital with the complaint of weakness of his right upper extremity. He couldn't use his hand at all. On this occasion there were definite neurological signs, and he was diagnosed as having a serious neuropathy (nerve disorder) affecting the hand and arm. Indeed, some wasting of muscles could already be noted. The somatic identification had forecast what area of his body would be affected.

ORIGINS

How does somatic identification get started? As infants we know the people in our lives only through our senses and through their satisfying our vital needs. Involved are the sight and voices of these key persons, their touching and holding us, and our associated body responses. It is as if we "introject" them, making them part of us in our primitive thoughts. Later in childhood, when we begin to speak and our ability to think develops, the original sensory impressions we have of those around us are replaced but not erased by ideas about them, ideas which are expressed by words. So that which very early in life is perceived as large, soft, warm, and a source of hunger relief becomes mother. But our sensory impressions of her never leave us.

So it is with other human beings with whom we have contact, and, of course, also with other objects. If relationships with our family are disturbed in childhood, we become aware of this at first through body sensations, subsequently through troubled thoughts and feelings. Later in life, should our dependency needs become activated and unfulfilled, or should be confronted with issues over control, competition, envy, or frustration of sexual longings, or with various unrealistic fears, we may regress, in varying degree and manner, to childhood patterns of response to stress. One way we then may adapt to the trouble confronting us is to become somewhat like the person whom we feel to be responsible for it. That person may be a member of our family or someone else who represents such a figure for us.

The more physical (sensory-motor-visceral) links there have been between us and such a family member, the greater the likelihood that our identification will reflect such physical elements. This is particularly true if that person has been ill or disabled during the time we were children. So, strange as it may seem, it is possible that someone who disturbs us emotionally may appear only briefly in our thoughts as such a person. But that is a sign of trouble, and subsequently we may become aware of discomfort in some part of our bodies. That bodily area has become a symbol of the person who upsets us. The existence of such sensitized areas or organs in us provides a target for physical disorder. Listen to yourself the next time you're talking about some part of your body that doesn't feel right. Are you referring to it as "he" or "she?"

LIKE THERAPIST, LIKE PATIENT

Here is an illustration of a patient in analysis having a physical reaction in a bodily area identical to one which was giving me trouble at the time. I represented a parental figure to him, and it was clear that he was identifying with me, the way I walked and the manner in which I spoke. Some months after he had begun treatment, I sustained an injury to the index finger of my left hand and had to have it splinted. When he made no mention of it for several days, I considered that a sign that some physical response in him would soon be evident. Finally, during an interview a week later, he did put his own hands behind his head, mentioning how much he had been biting his nails and calling my attention to an infection in his right middle finger. The next day the patient finally mentioned my splinted finger, wondering if I had cut it or had infected it as had happened to him. He felt it served me right because I was not taking care of his emotional needs. Again, he stopped making references to my injury. This was suggestive that more might happen to him physically. Then he missed an appointment because of a cold and, when he returned, belittled himself for staying out. He had had a brief but severe spasm of his larynx and thought he would choke to death. After that, his internist started him on antibiotics. On resuming the interviews, the patient recalled that during his childhood his father had had many sore throats. He again clasped his hands behind his head. He then pointedly asked if I could see two red, swollen areas on his left hand. One was located on the back of his left index finger (same finger involved as mine), and the other was lower down on the hand. His physician had called it an allergic reaction to the antibiotics.

So identification sometimes assumes physical forms. When we are under stress, thinking about the people with whom our relationships are strained, especially about their illnesses (past and present, if any), provides indications of which organ or organ system in our bodies may be affected or what kind of illness may develop in us.

Actions Dangerous to Health

Besides affecting our bodies directly, emotion can do so indirectly by first influencing our *behavior*. Then, if our actions are neurotic, we may expose ourselves to harmful situations and increase our chances of becoming disabled and ill.

BEHAVIORAL GUIDELINES

What forecasts the likelihood of such an outcome? First, there is a tendency for some of us to act more and think less. We respond to stress by giving very little thought to it; instead we behave ("act out") in ways that often can hurt us. Second and related is the impulsiveness involved in such behavior. The roots of impulsive behavior go back to early childhood when we tolerated delay of physical and emotional gratification least well. If we don't outgrow this intolerance, then later frustration of our needs will push us toward overly quick and often inappropriate behavior. At times, strong desires to which our conscience and reason both say no may become so compelling that we disregard the voices of caution and act impulsively. Though we know that no good will come of our behavior, we cannot stop, and then it leads us straight to harm, often involving our bodies.

But conflict can occur when we feel compelled to act immediately, possibly violently, and try at the same time to restrain our impulses lest we be rejected by family and friends. If we find ourselves caught in such an unresolved struggle, it, too, is a sign that tensions are building up, that adequate psychological outlets are blocked and that our bodies can become targets. In still another way, behavior which is ingratiating and inappropriate, calculated to interest others in us so we'll not feel utterly rejected and defective, becomes a sign of possible trouble when it backfires and does not get us what we crave. Then we're left hurting, and the repercussions could affect our bodies.

Our behavior is determined by a mixture of rational, conscious thought plus *irrational* impulses whose meaning is mostly outside our awareness. Though our unconscious motives usually predominate over our more sensible thinking, the indicators outlined above are useful warnings that our behavior may do us in. This is not to say that we can always avoid unhealthy situations. Poverty, crime, slums, overcrowding, simple ignorance, and other hard realities condemn many of us to be trapped in environments which breed disease. I am referring to harmful exposure that can be avoided, if we can recognize that emotional forces are driving us there and if we can divert them.

ACTIVISTS VS. THINKERS

Let's consider what may happen to people who tend to act more and think less: people who are impulsive. When they are faced by urgent needs, they don't stop to figure out the best course of action, and this gets them into trouble. Let's say you're such a person and you've lost a close relative or a dear friend; or a love affair has ended badly. You feel drained, alone. If you're inclined to be headstrong and to act quickly, you might look for a way out of your depression without thinking things through. You've heard certain drugs make you feel real happy. So because your impulsiveness has shut your judgment off, you buy those drugs without thinking of the consequences—and are amazed to find yourself freaking out or becoming an addict. Or suppose you've had a violent quarrel, feel you've been given a raw deal. You act fast, get into your car, race away over the speed limit, and crash, winding up in the hospital badly injured. Or perhaps you're a dignified professional man, married, with homosexual tendencies. You're so frustrated in your sexual relations with your wife that, before sober thought can intervene, you pick up a willing young man in a public toilet and persuade him to let you suck his erect penis. Three weeks later a syphilitic chancre marks the spot in your mouth. In all of these cases you're paying with a vengeance for your rashness.

These are, of course, extreme examples. But we adults *do* punish ourselves in many lesser ways even if we aren't aware of what this behavior means because, strange as it sounds, punishment can bring some sense of relief. Under what circumstances? When there is deeply hidden guilt which plagues us until we have atoned in some measure for it. It's a holdover from childhood when, if we had forbidden fantasies or our wishes were not fulfilled, we would act in a naughty way and *that* could lead to being spanked. Even if it hurt, we felt relieved afterward; at least our bad conscience would stop tormenting us for a while. Though we don't seek to hurt ourselves consciously, we may even become "accident-prone," that is, we let our unconscious impulses lead us to danger without being able to use the resources of our common sense to save ourselves. This happens when we are riddled with guilt, even though most of it is irrational.

RENDEZVOUS WITH DEATH

Consider these more detailed examples. Mort, who had spoiled his kid rotten, felt uneasy and tense as he settled into the plane on his way back home from still another talk with this only son. The kid wasn't getting anywhere. He wanted to drop out of college despite the nice apartment Mort had set him up in. "There was something terrible about the way I brought the kid up," Mort thought to himself. "I overindulged him, gave him his own way all the time." Mort wanted the boy to get all the breaks he had never had, coming from a big family, just barely existing during the Depression years, never thinking about himself but working like hell to get to be a partner in a construction company. Now the kid was going to have to see a psychiatrist. That's what all the kids at school were doing—going to shrinks. *What* had he done wrong?

As the plane took off, Mort discovered his friend Flexy was aboard. Mort didn't feel like talking, but he also wanted everyone to like him; so he let Flexy kid him until he actually forgot his troubles. Had he really forgotten? Or would his troubled conscience reassert itself in some other way? When they landed, Mort was going to head for the subway, but Flexy would have none of that: "Look, it's raining, and I've got my car here. I'll drop you off at a cab stand in town." Mort wanted to refuse—the subway would really be faster —but he couldn't bring himself to say no. He was too afraid of offending a friend. So he reluctantly let Flexy drop him off at a cab stand, but the only taxi there pulled out as he approached. In an increasingly black mood in the cold rain, Mort headed across some tracks toward a streetcar stop, and he kept right on even when he heard a streetcar coming. As he touched the slippery rails, his legs suddenly gave out under him. He slipped and fell under the onrushing wheels.

Why had Mort become careless? Because he felt so miserable, he no longer tried to protect himself or to exercise reasonable caution. He thought he had failed as a parent. Nobody seemed to care about him. And to top everything, he had let Flexy lead him around like a puppy. His harsh conscience had always taken him to task for even little mistakes. Usually when it was bothering him, he would torment himself over everything he had ever done wrong, or thought was wrong, and he would feel depressed. Sometimes to cover up his moodiness, he would pretend to be extra friendly, as he had with Flexy. But he always got mad at himself later, because by pretending everything was fine he ended up suffering more. So then he would act out—would express his anger by getting back at himself for being so stupid—by kicking at some furniture or even by depriving himself of a good time. Falling under the streetcar was in accord with an old pattern of self-punishment mostly achieved through self-destructive behavior, but this time the need for it had accumulated to a point of overwhelming intensity without his being aware that this was happening.

This is the danger of falling into a pattern where we constantly *behave* in such a way as to inflict little punishments on ourselves. Banging our fists on a table or wall is a relatively harmless release when we are momentarily angry. But it does little good to use it over and over to try to relieve the intense feelings of deprivation, frustration, or anger over nobody's caring about us. These build up within us and we are impelled to *act* in ways that hurt us more and more until, like Mort, we can do ourselves in.

AN IMPULSIVE INVESTOR BLEEDS

Here is another example. After still one more quarrel with his wife, Vesterow thought the marriage was all over.

It was the same thing: her sarcasm and her devaluation of him. It was all about money—the way he insisted on managing the savings of twenty years. He kept thinking it was *his* money and he had earned it—every penny. They were comfortably off; the education for the kids was all taken care of; there was plenty of insurance. What more did his wife want? Vesterow, furious, vowed to change his wife's mind about him. More than that, he was going to get even with her. (Little Big Shot was her favorite expression for him, and at times she made it sound like something else.)

Vesterow was rarely rash. In fact, he was rather compulsive by nature, thinking everything through very carefully, to the last detail. Yet every once in a great while, he reacted the opposite way, with impulsive behavior, and it was usually after a big scene between himself and his wife, when his feelings of being unwanted and unappreciated would reach a high pitch. The impulsiveness was known to him, but he disregarded the sign that he might do something he would regret on this day. As he sat in the board room, distraught, with the quarrel ringing in his ears, Vesterow stared at the moving tape and decided he would get back at his wife by making a killing. She wouldn't give him any support or consideration; well, he'd get it for himself from the market. And he'd show her he was somebody after all. The averages had been going up. But the one stock into which he had sunk fifteen thousand dollars remained annoyingly static. No change. Just like his ulcer. Status quo. Vesterow had been following his doctor's advice: Bland diet, antacids, some tranquilizers.

An uneasy feeling in the pit of his stomach intruded as he recalled the name of a highly touted, speculative stock he would normally have laughed at. Now a curious debate began to develop in Vesterow's mind. Plunge—be careful. Take a chance—can't afford to. Terrific profits—don't believe it. A voice of caution kept interfering with his fantasies.

Back and forth the argument went. Suddenly, *impulsively,* Vesterow traded his solid stock for the speculative one. The debate had ended, in favor of gambling to become a rich somebody. Fantasies of triumph stilled the voice of caution so completely that despite his ulcer Vesterow decided to celebrate with a drink. One bourbon and ginger ale wouldn't hurt. And it didn't. But he spent more and more time watching the tape, and taking one "careful" drink a day, and the uneasiness in his stomach got worse as his speculative venture went nowhere.

Then one morning his new stock opened weak and proceeded to decline relentlessly. Vesterow skipped lunch. His horror, his disgust with himself for not heeding the voice of caution, and feelings of helplessness grew as the stock continued to dip. Just before the closing bell, Vesterow's fifteen thousand dollars had shrunk to three thousand. He could no longer pretend he had not been crap-shooting against his better judgment. His stomach felt like an iron knot, twisting and turning. At the bar he half-spilled the first highball, his hands were shaking so badly. It did nothing for him. He managed to get down all of a second drink. When the waitress asked if he wanted a refill, he stared at her. Then, instead of words, a geyser of blood erupted from his mouth all over the front of her pretty uniform.

Anxiety, depression, and anger—the product of his impulsive behavior which was thinly covered over by fantastic hopes of a kill—had done him in. Always before, his stomach had been a target for assaults from his inner tensions. Yet he had known this and had been careful to heed his doctor's advice. Now it was once again taking the major impact of the enormous mental strain he had been under. And this time, instead of protecting his body, he had allowed his rage and worry to make him act impulsively. That produced more tension, which led him to alcohol. And the alcohol, in turn, doubled the insult to his vulnerable stomach. Its lining, always irritated when *he* was irritated, now had been eaten away by acid in one spot, eroding a small blood vessel. The diagnosis at the hospital was bleeding peptic ulcer. Only quick transfusions saved Vesterow's life.

Most of us like to think we are a little more careful than Mort, and we wouldn't try to cross tracks in front of an oncoming streetcar on a dark, rainy night. Yet the truth is that, like Vesterow, we can also put ourselves in jeopardy by *not* acting in our own best interests and doing it in a less direct and more gradual way.

THE RECKLESS NURSE

A third instance of how disturbed emotions signal that they may relentlessly lead us into a harmful situation is Miss Darren's case. An experienced practical nurse who had made many visits in high-crime areas, her actions one early winter evening were irrational. Having completed a home visit in one of the worst sections of the city, she refused the offer of her patient's husband to walk her to the subway or to a cab. That, in itself was unusual. She certainly knew that an unescorted woman was courting danger. Normally she would not have been so careless. But of late, Miss Darren had been feeling—well, she couldn't quite make out whether she was bored or depressed or both. She was in her late thirties and, thinking her chances of getting a man were rapidly diminishing, she had clutched at a new doctor at the clinic. But the relationship went nowhere in a hurry. All he offered was some sex and nothing else, and Miss Darren had been feeling let down for weeks now. She was also troubled about her two brothers, one of whom she thought had been neglecting her, and the other of whom she had not seen recently even though he had developed asthma. Preoccupied, she had chosen to be alone with her thoughts rather than with the safety of a companion.

As she hurried down the narrow, deserted street, a bulky

form suddenly stepped out from the doorway of the rotting, empty house and struck her a glancing blow on the head. She stumbled, and another blow knocked her to her knees. She was unable even to whisper as panic and the blows numbed her brain. The attacker, a powerful man, dragged her into the unlit hallway and struck her again. Waves of nausea rocked her and she felt utterly helpless. Her coat was torn off, her dress ripped. Big hands pawed her, pulling at her brassiere, and then her panties. No strength to fight back. Only a dull question: Will he kill me? In the dark she could not see the man's face. And then that was over. When he got up, there was a knife in his hand. But a couple of giggling teenagers burst into the hallway, and he fled past them.

Miss Darren had come close to paying in full because of her irrational behavior. Her emotional upset had made her blind to physical danger. Ironically, the punishment that befell her far exceeded the guilt that had been troubling her.

In many instances, irrational behavior similarly leads us into situations which may be directly or indirectly harmful. Adolescents, for example, are often goaded or encouraged by gangs or groups of friends to court physical trouble by the use of drugs, by insufficient and inadequate diet, poor hygiene, unsanitary food and water, or by promiscuity resulting in venereal disease or in pregnancy and abortion. To be sure, you can take chances without any dramatic, severe, or long-lasting effects. But so often we bring illness on ourselves or otherwise damage our bodies simply because we haven't taken reasonable precautions.

That's why we cannot quickly dismiss so-called careless behavior. One thing that Mort, Vesterow, and Miss Darren have in common with so many of us is an inability, and often an unwillingness, to examine all motives before acting. We should try to do this *particularly* if we are troubled and confused about whether our behavior is realistic or impulsive. At the least, we can ask ourselves whether we tend to act on impulse and have gotten into trouble before because of that, whether we're easily frustrated, whether our strict conscience drives us to dangerous extremes.

AVOIDANCE OF PSEUDO-DANGER

We have been discussing how emotion makes us disregard danger and hurt ourselves unnecessarily. Let us now consider an opposite kind of behavior. This consists of avoiding things or situations whose dangerous possibilities are exaggerated *far* beyond reality. For instance, some people are terrified of heights; even though they are nowhere near the edge of the high spot (upper story, roof, cliff), they are petrified of falling. Others refuse to drive, afraid they will lose control over the car. Still others refuse to ride in a car they are not operating because they have *no* control over it. Many avoid trains, planes, and boats for similar reasons. There are people who cannot tolerate even a speck of dirt because they believe it will lead to infection. Such unusual fears are called phobias—there are many different kinds—and the people who experience them are phobic. One very common condition in which these manifestations occur is motion sickness (even on a merry-go-round). Phobic persons are not really afraid of heights, cars, planes, boats, etc. Their anxiety evolves from the fact that such objects have for them a symbolic, irrational meaning of something dangerous and forbidden, either a sexual or aggressive impulse, which can lead to unpleasant consequences. If they are afraid of high places, they are probably concerned about the rising sexual excitement they experience in such locations. They won't ride on trains, planes, or boats because they believe it will be impossible to get out in an emergency and that thought is unbearable. Actually it represents a disguised fear that they will lose control of erotic or aggressive wishes that can be stirred up in them by the constant sensation of motion. If they are overly concerned about germs, they are really anxious about "dirty impulses" (which the germs symbolize) lurking deep within them. And so on. The end result of such fears is quite sad, since phobic people in their attempts to avoid anxiety isolate themselves from other people and restrict their activities more and more.

If you are a classic phobic and force yourself or are forced into a feared situation, that is a signal that you will probably develop troublesome physical symptoms such as nausea, dizziness, or fainting, but these are manifestations of anxiety rather than physical disease.

However, there are all degrees of anxiety about heights, flying, germs, etc., so that we do not necessarily have to be considered phobic if we are under tension in these particular situations. And simple anxiety-relieving measures are then sufficient to calm us down and make us more comfortable—for example, a word of reassurance from someone we trust; absorption in an interesting conversation; or a mild tranquilizing tablet.

It would be most useful to determine which fears make sense and protect our well-being, and which are simply so ridiculous and abnormal that they restrict our lives unnecessarily. This may seem a hard decision, since a full enjoyment of life means taking some risks. Nevertheless, in many instances a sane balance is not so difficult to achieve if we give our actions forethought. A good example might be swimming, which can add fun and relaxation to our lives. Should the fact that people drown deter us? The answer would be no, if we swim in safe water within our capabilities. Yet people, driven either by a need for self-punishment or a need to prove they are not anxious and fearful types, disregard the posted warnings, the real dangers, and expose themselves to injury or death. So, when we are faced with any other action we might or might not take, it will help to keep in mind that intolerance of tension and attempts to escape from emotional troubles through impulsive behavior may lead us straight to physical disability.

PART THREE

*Some
Applications
of
Psychological
Prediction*

12

Nervous Pounds of Flesh

Obesity is the reason why as many as ten million persons in this country seek medical advice every year. Dozens of books have been written about this condition; hundreds of diets and billions of assorted pills have been prescribed to treat it. The focus has been on physical aspects, while the role of emotional factors in obesity continues to be controversial or lightly passed over. My intention is not to debate what the most likely causes or best cures of weight problems are, but to show that psychological signs can warn us when these difficulties are likely to develop or recur. Knowing about such indicators will help us prevent obesity, or malnutrition, and if either has already become established, will help predict any worsening of the condition.

IN THE BEGINNING—ALL MOUTH

As infants we use our mouths not only for eating, but to satisfy sucking needs which are a very early form of our emotional needs. An infant puts everything it can into its mouth—fingers, pacifiers, blankets, toys—and this interest in our mouths is something we never quite get over. As older children, even as grown-ups, we suck our thumbs, bite our nails, run fingers and pencils over our lips, chew gum, and otherwise keep our mouths busy. That always indicates that we feel a need for some quick emotional gratification, which we try to give ourselves through such activities.

Though a baby sees, hears, smells, and touches, he (or she) also uses his mouth to explore and make contact with the world around him. To an infant, the mother's breast, a bottle, the milk—even the mother—are all one. Being fed, cuddled, rocked, mothered are all simple ways he understands he's being loved. If he isn't fed fast enough, doesn't get enough sucking and mothering, if these "oral needs" are insufficiently gratified, he gets mad—crying, twisting his body, and making mouth movements. When he gets really upset, he may refuse food even if he's hungry, or vomit it up after forced feeding.

Gradually the baby does begin to realize that the things around him—breast, bottle, mother—are different, separate objects. By then he is so involved in handling things, learning to walk, learning to talk, that his mouth is ordinarily no longer so important. Yet he never gets over the feeling that being fed and being loved are closely linked even though, as he grows older, such a thought rises less and less to his conscious mind. This "oral" phase (of getting emotional satisfaction), if it is marked by unusual frustration or over-gratification, can persist to such an extent that it interferes with normal development. The fixation often adversely affects our body functions and particularly our eating habits in childhood or later in life, as we shall see.

ADULT PACIFIERS

As adults we eat at mealtimes, usually unaware that we are satisfying our "oral needs" as well as our stomachs. If we also need snacks, sodas, candy, or anything to chew on between meals, we don't pay much attention to these as emotional supplements either. And so we fail to realize that, if we indulge our mouths too much, it is a sign that we have never quite outgrown that babylike state in which our mouths are all-important—that we are stuffing our mouths as a holdover from the days when being fed meant we were loved.

Thus, as adults, we turn eating, smoking, or chewing on a pencil into a comfort, a pacifier to relieve emotional stress, without being aware of the significance of this behavior. Such actions are signs that we are releasing some little tensions in us; here indulgence in orality acts as a safety valve. However, when we try to use mouth activity to release great troubles and worries, we're on our way to creating more rather than fewer problems for ourselves. If we eat too much or smoke, our pacifiers may turn out to be as harmful as the internal turmoil we are trying to remedy.

Specifically, those of us who gain too much weight may have felt emotionally deprived and unloved in childhood—and stuffed ourselves on food then (as we do now) because we associated it with the comfort and warmth of our baby days. Our distraught parents were probably so worried over getting us to eat "properly" that they overlooked the fact that we felt starved for affection and attention. Failure to recognize such emotional deprivation in children (revealed in their play, fantasies, and dreams) is failure to recognize a sign that points to the likely development of eating troubles then or later. Childhood is a critical time for preventing such conditions from developing because, once established, they are difficult to modify.

CHILDHOOD LINKS

So, when we are children, parental or sibling attitudes toward food can indicate what our own eating habits will be. Our parents may have placed too much emphasis on food, believing that a hefty child is a healthy one, and forcing us to eat too much. If they themselves were overweight, we also might have identified with them and automatically assumed we should be overweight too. Perhaps at mealtimes our parents threatened, "I won't love you if you don't eat your vegetables (or take your vitamins, or clean up your plate)." Perhaps they rewarded us for "good" behavior by offering fattening sweets—ice cream, cookies, or chocolate. These early experiences can stay with us in adulthood. Awareness of such conditioning and our tendency to associate food with emotional satisfactions should be a warning to us that an eating splurge is in the offing when we are subjected to great emotional pressures. So we gain weight if we ignore the signs that we need relief from our tensions—past as well as present—because we will try to get this relief by overeating instead of seeking it through counseling or therapy.

Pressuring children to eat can cause food to become overly important to them in two particular ways, each of which can lead to trouble. They may either comply or rebel—stuff themselves, or go to the opposite extreme of pecking at their food. A lot depends on what goes on during mealtime. How the family sits around the dining table is usually not just chance, but reflects the relationships among members of the family. Father, at the head of the table, is demonstrating his authority. Mother, at the foot, is subservient and silent. The children are not to speak unless spoken to. That's one model. A patient of mine described how his gadgeteer father dealt with six noisy boys at family dinner—by using a wooden knuckle rapper at the end of a rod. Without having to get up or say a word, he could rap the knuckles of any child getting out of hand.

Maybe Mother spends all of the dinner hour showing she's boss, or both parents argue, or the children are free to be unruly. A chair next to Father and Mother may signify favoritism. Seating may be changed to reward or punish the children. An only child may find himself in between two adults in more ways than one. Some families exclude the younger children from eating with the rest of the group, perhaps until they have learned to behave like little adults, and that point of grace may vary considerably in each family.

Mealtime may be formal or informal, varying with the time of day or specialness of the occasion. It may be hurried or dragged out. The kitchen, dining room, or "family room" may be the site. Television-watching may silence all eaters. Mealtime may openly and loudly reflect the tensions of the day, or be a time for happy conversation.

In any event, the kind of things talked about, the specific interchanges between father and mother, between parents and children, between children and children, the various rewards and punishments meted out at the dining table all contribute to the symbolic meaning that eating has for us.

GOURMET

Let's see how this played a role in Dolores' life when she was twenty-two. She thought of herself as a career girl, but really wanted to get married. Her latest boyfriend, a medical student, seemed a likely prospect. The evening before his last and most important exam, when she suggested they go out to eat, he agreed. After dinner, Dolores, mindful of his exam, wanted to go back to the apartment. Strangely, he insisted on lingering over after-dinner liqueurs. So they got home late, and he stayed up even later studying.

The next morning he went into a panic about the exam and, out of the blue, accused her of not being considerate of him. After a furious few minutes, he stomped out. She was stunned. The attack was uncalled-for. He could have refused to eat out. And why had he dawdled in the restaurant when she had insisted on leaving early so he could study? It was unfair. She felt terribly criticized and rejected. Suddenly a crazy idea hit her; she thought she was fifty pounds overweight and almost as obese as her parents and sister. She rushed to the full-length mirror in the bedroom. She wasn't that heavy at all, her eyes told her. She got on the scale. Just a few pounds above what was the best weight for her. But there was no feeling of relief. Instead she began to feel deprived and hollow.

This gyration from a sensation of heaviness to one of emptiness, from thinking herself overweight to thinking herself starved, was a sign that she would turn to food for consolation. She barely controlled the impulse to stuff herself. That night she dreamed—to her it seemed endlessly—about being the empress of a faraway country and being waited on hand and foot, her every desire anticipated and fulfilled. When she awoke the dream haunted her for hours. It was, in fact, another sign of things to come.

For the next few days she and her boyfriend tried to patch things up. When he left for a visit with his parents, Dolores seemed calm, but her behavior signaled that her emotional needs continued to be great. She bought herself a cookbook, a fancy one, and embarked on a cooking spree, compulsively making exotic delicacies for herself. No stuffing, but really unusual dishes.

What had Dolores' earlier life been like? Why was making a fuss over food her way of trying to calm her tension? As a child she had been very thin, in striking contrast to her obese sister and parents. Her father at one time was sixty pounds overweight, but after dieting he lost almost forty pounds (though he seemed shrunken after that). Her mother weighed over two hundred pounds, the heaviest of them all. She was a night eater, starting early in the evening and nibbling away well into the late hours. The oddest part was that the father did all the cooking and shopping. He was boss of the kitchen. And he made rules. Nobody, wife or children, could have the last of any food in the refrigerator. A small portion always had to be left, and that was reserved for him. He also did other strange things. He took to hiding small caches of goodies all over the house, so that nobody else could get at them. Nuts of various kinds were a favorite item, and these were stored in secret hiding places. The family nicknamed him "the Squirrel."

Dolores knew it was all rather weird, but she'd never tried to figure it out. However, these early experiences had had a profound influence on her. Neither of her parents ever gave her much attention or love. As a child she felt repelled by their obesity, but later in life she herself turned secretly to food when other sources could not supply the affection she had missed in her childhood. And her need to be loved had led her to overreact to this latest incident.

Instead of realizing that her boyfriend had just been so nervous over his exam that he'd become unreasonable, she was afraid of losing him. The criticism that she was inconsiderate had come across as "You're too greedy." And that had made her feel temporarily that she was being accused of wanting to devour everything. That's why she had the illusion that she was fat, until the mirror and scales convinced her otherwise. Nevertheless she felt compelled to favor herself, to give herself special things (in the form of food) to make up for her getting no satisfaction on her job and also for her possibly losing her boyfriend. To a certain extent she was behaving like her father. Not stuffing herself, but controlling her emotional upset through special foods.

For many of us food and the comfort from eating can relieve tension, but it is not a good way. A signal of things to come is that if we eat to feel better, we'll eat even more, hoping to feel even better—until finally no amount of food may be sufficient.

THE ADS ADD

Excessive preoccupation with appearance is another sign that problems with food are likely. Suppose we have a craving for food, but from all sides—television, movies, newspapers, magazines, and billboards—the virtues of the slim, trim figure for women and the athletic, muscular physique for men are extolled and made into status symbols. How do we resolve the dilemma? Some highly suggestible people go to extraordinary extremes. They gorge themselves with food, then make themselves vomit, thus seemingly satisfying both the need to eat and the wish to be slim. Or they diet and diet and are always hungry and irritable.

In addition to the barrages about how we should look, we are also bombarded by warnings of how fat people will have heart attacks, strokes, and other illnesses. Being fat may become a constant source of anxiety, partly realistic, partly irrational, and ironically the worry itself sometimes can prove more damaging to us than the fat.

It's common sense to say extremes of all kinds are best avoided, and that applies to eating and dieting. Trying to look like the beautiful people is an exercise in neurotic futility, stemming chiefly from feelings of inferiority. Relaxation of inner tensions and achievement of reasonably good health are much better reasons for dealing with weight problems. In any case, their solution should be attempted under expert guidance which takes into consideration *both* emotional and physical makeup.

FOOD AGAINST SEX

Extremes of weight are predictable when we find ourselves using our appearance as an excuse for avoiding certain social, physical, or sexual activities. For instance, men with doubts about their sexual prowess may turn to incessant eating. They become so fat that they have no sex appeal and no longer feel obligated to prove their masculinity in this way. Women who don't enjoy sexual activity may either gorge or starve themselves to become so unattractive that men lose interest in them; then they no longer have to worry about getting sexually involved.

An example of why a woman might turn to such an odd defense might be a traumatic love affair. Take Lois, a twenty-seven-year-old executive secretary—pretty, vivacious, and a virgin. Though she tended to gain weight, she was usually successful in keeping her figure trim as long as she followed a diet. She had dated on and off in a desultory way but now was harboring a secret crush on her boss, an older, married man who was not unaware of her interest in him. At the office Christmas party they began to flirt in earnest, and her boss finally offered to drive her home. They parked and petted for a while, but Lois became afraid that her sexual excitement would lead to intercourse. She refused to participate any further. On the way to her apartment her boss stopped for more drinks. When they started up again he was quite drunk but insisted on driving. A short time later he crashed into a telephone pole and was instantly killed, while Lois escaped with cuts and bruises.

The following weeks were a prolonged nightmare. She felt guilty and ashamed. A short vacation did not help. Neither did changing her job. She remained depressed. She tried to stop herself from constantly reliving the crash in her mind, but for a while could not. She dreamed of accidents and awoke screaming. Then it all suddenly disappeared from her thoughts and dreams. Her tortured feelings subsided. She seemed mysteriously calm. In effect, a shift in her emotional equilibrium had taken place, reflected in dreams of being a child who was adored by her parents, and of presiding over sumptuous feasts. That was an indication of things to come. Her appetite improved remarkably. Sweets, especially banana splits, provided more relief from tension than tranquilizers. Gradually her desire for such goodies became insatiable. As she gobbled more and more sweets, she seemed almost happy, and her depression did not return. When she was a child, her father had often told her how pretty she was but kept reminding her he didn't like her tendency to get plump. She resembled her mother, a pretty but obese woman who ate whenever she was unhappy, who was uninterested in sex, and who didn't get along well with her husband. He was an executive in his father-in-law's business, a position which he was reluctant to give up and which tied him to the marriage. So the unhappy couple was stuck with each other, and the little girl was buffeted by their emotional storms. They often quarreled openly, and sometimes there was physical violence which Lois witnessed.

Because of her mother's interest in food, there was always an overflowing larder. As a child, Lois automatically ate and ate, trying to fill the void in her, especially when she felt her parents were too busy with their troubles to pay attention to her. And that was often enough. And she could get her mother's attention that way—even her praise. During brief intervals of calm, the mother gave big parties, feeding lots of people. Those were the moments when the obese woman was least troubled. People thought her a most gracious hostess, and her daughter got the idea that big feasts made people happy.

So as a little girl Lois had developed not only a craving for food, but a strong impression that married life was hell. She came to regard men, beginning with her father, as difficult to please, even violent. As she grew up, this uneasiness and distrust lingered, though she tried to cover it up with a façade of gaiety. It seemed natural to do as her mother had done—indulge herself with food, especially sweets, when she felt that life was treating her badly. It was therefore no surprise that Lois would use this familiar way to deal with the troublesome memories of her recent affair. And she didn't pay any more attention to men. They, in turn, soon stopped paying her much attention either, as her body got fatter and fatter. Lois had escaped physical illness, but not without paying a price.

NIGHT EATERS

About ten percent of obese people have no appetite in the morning and afternoon, but are voracious night-time eaters. Once they start eating in the evening, they consume larger and larger amounts of food at shorter and shorter intervals. As the evening progresses, eating becomes practically nonstop. Many of these people are chronically depressed, though they usually have no awareness of what conflicts are involved. Any increase in depression is a signal that a food orgy is likely. They start off the day feeling so blue they can't eat. Toward evening a psychological shift occurs and they react in an opposite way—they try to cope with the empty feeling by filling up with food. Once the eating starts, it rapidly builds up to an incredible pitch.

A WAY OF LIFE

Thus, those of us who are dissatisfied, lonely, frustrated, or disappointed may derive some emotional relief from eating. In some cases, moreover, eating may even assume a *primary* place in our lives. Phil Rupp's case is typical. Phil spent day after tiring day doing the same old thing at the gas station. Taking the crap from customers and his boss. A passive man stuck in a rut and sinking deeper into it every year. Lots of cokes and cigarettes during the day. He couldn't wait to get back to his little apartment. For what? Not women. Dates had become infrequent. He was getting into the late thirties, and besides, women cost too much. Those were the arguments he gave himself, arguments that covered up feelings of inferiority and doubts about his manliness. No, he had a huge TV screen and a very comfortable armchair, and he spent most evenings with his eyes glued to the set, jaws crunching. It wasn't the taste of the food so much as the muscles working away that gave him a peculiar sense of satisfaction. And also the chewing, the swallowing, the lifting of hand to mouth, of bottle to mouth. He had a compulsion to keep opening the refrigerator. Phil was an "oral person," a heritage from a very unhappy childhood when he fought with his brothers over food, of which there never seemed to be enough. He always got the worst of everything.

In that chair, taking in everything he could—with his eyes and his mouth—he was simply obeying all the ads that encouraged him to eat or drink something or to smoke cigars (for extra pleasure, and to enhance your manliness and attract the chicks). And to further blot out reality, he could identify with the hero and win the heroine in the rerun movies. So Phil had given up trying to make friends, have a relationship, or do anything else—until finally life meant only a TV screen and food.

FAT IS NOT HAPPY

Is the happy, fat person really happy? Not necessarily and not often. It is common for fat people who are always clowning to be miserable underneath. *Extremes of feeling or behavior are often signs that the very opposite is being warded off.* Merivale made lots of people laugh and even cry a little. He played the comic with just the right touch of pathos. Although short and fat, he could really fit into many roles—the slob bumbling in and out of trouble; the arrogant man who said the most outrageous things (the sheer hostility made you laugh in relief because someone else had dared voice what was in your mind); the tricky conniver who always was found out and, after confessing, was forgiven.

But even though he made audiences laugh, after each performance he would retire into loneliness except for a faithful valet—and then he would eat. He could afford the most expensive food and drink and did not stint. That was the kind of life, the kind of balance he had maintained for years. It was a defense against a bottomless void in his feelings and also against the likelihood of a breakdown.

Nobody knew his background, because he never mentioned his past. When he had become successful, he had plucked his senile folks out of the slums and stashed them away in a home for the elderly somewhere in the sticks. He rarely visited them. The check, however, was sent regularly. All he could remember of his childhood was that both parents were constantly drunk and beat him if he went near them. So he had run away when he was a kid, bummed around for years—always hungry, ragged, and lousy—in and out of the lockup for vagrancy. But his own misery had led him to be keenly aware of other people's suffering, their dreams of glory, the many absurdities of life around him. And he had talent. He could make people laugh, even tough hoboes and tough cops. That talent gradually ripened; he finally got some breaks, began to make money, and left the old life behind him. No more wanting a decent meal. But now, no matter how much he ate, he still felt hungry. A topnotch performer, a money-maker, a success, he felt emotionally starved. Except for his valet, he hardly saw other people outside working hours. Underneath that exterior that made thousands laugh, there was depression.

One night he was in the middle of an eating orgy, surrounded by the finest foods, when the phone rang. There had been a fire. Both his parents had been burned to death.

Merivale had hated his parents, wanted them out of the way—but not *completely* out of the way. He thought he had put them away *safely*, because often, secretly, he had pictured them as different, he had dreamed of another kind of childhood, kept hoping they would show signs that they really had cared about him. Now they were gone.

For a few days he couldn't forget them or forgive himself. He suffered from melancholia and self-recrimination, stopped eating, and finally felt blank, numb. The apathy was a signal that a long-standing emotional equilibrium had been upset in him and that trouble was brewing.

Then he began to eat again, more voraciously than ever. It was a desperate effort to take the edge off his almost intolerable depression. Finally he became so huge he could hardly move. Only when his livelihood was threatened by his inability to get around did he finally seek professional help. The first specialist found nothing wrong physically and prescribed a strict diet. Merivale lost some weight but couldn't keep up the diet and went back to stuffing himself. The second specialist prescribed some pills, another diet, and exercises. He urged Merivale to use willpower. Again the results were discouraging. The third doctor wanted to learn something about Merivale's personal life. It was no easy matter to talk about things that had been kept hidden for a lifetime, but Merivale was determined to go through with the treatment. Ever so gradually he began to understand how his hunger and depression, his attempts to cope with loneliness by gorging himself, had roots reaching back into his troubled childhood and adolescence. And he saw how the death of his parents had triggered off a severe upset in which his guilt threatened to overwhelm him. As his insight into his hangups increased, his emotional starvation became less troublesome. Therapy was long and difficult, but Merivale stuck it out and his story had a happy ending.

His experience and that of many others underscores the fact that it's better not to wait until we get into a jam with overeating before seeking help for the tensions associated with it. Early consultation, when emotional signs warn us we're on the brink, may prevent a lot of complications, both mental *and* physical, later on.

STARVATION AND MALNUTRITION

As we have seen, for many, many people, eating is not just a matter of nutrition, it is also a way of getting comfort for emotional hurts—and a way of defending against depression or physical illness. On the other hand, there are people who stop eating when they feel very upset. And some react both ways (gluttony followed by starvation) when they feel abandoned. Let's see what happened to Laura when she and her boyfriend had their big argument. When were they going to get married? Sooner, she said. Later, he said. Besides, he wanted her to lose some weight. That last remark upset her so much she found it hard to think straight. Heaviness had always been a sore point with this woman.

When she was little and the kids called her "fatty," she got so mad she sometimes bit them. She'd get beaten for that, so she gave it up, though she never got over the urge to bite when she got angry. She learned to bite on hard food instead, or to grind her teeth together (a common expression of anger many of us share at times). At times she felt sad and did not eat at all, which aroused her parents' concern.

Laura dieted listlessly from time to time as she grew up, but without success. Outwardly, she seemed to accept what she called her fate, but pain and bitterness seethed inside her when anyone commented on her appearance. It was a sure indication that eventually she would lose control, and that's what happened this time. She burst into tears and disappeared into the kitchen. She came back munching on a carrot, a celery stick, another carrot. The argument continued. Back into the kitchen. This time it was an apple, another apple, a hunk of hard chocolate. The chomping jaws reflected her frustration at not being able to control her fatness and her anger at her boyfriend for bringing it up. Her suffering silence gained nothing; her boyfriend walked out in disgust.

The next night, she was alone. That's when her binge began. Uncontrollable eating. All the next day and well into the night. Everything in sight. Again, as she had done in childhood, afraid of being abandoned and feeling empty, she stuffed herself. Eating helped calm her, and she emerged from the panic; her thoughts became clearer. She was shocked that her anger had been so intense she had actually wanted to kill her boyfriend. Her conscience began to trouble her. She groped for a way out of the mess, and a "solution" finally occurred to her. She would show him she *could* become thin. She was about to shift from one extreme to another in her eating behavior and was unaware that this could endanger her health.

She began to starve herself—an extreme diet with insufficient fluid intake. Several times she was so panicked at the idea of staying fat that, even though she had eaten little, she made herself vomit by sticking a finger in her throat. Her weight dropped and dropped. Then she developed a small cold. But her body's powers of resistance had become dangerously depressed by starvation and emotional shock. The cold bloomed into pneumonia, and she had to be hospitalized. Skillful medical attention saved her life. There was a bonus, ironically—a sickbed reconciliation with her boyfriend. But the price had almost been too great.

Dieting, self-prescribed, based on what relatives, friends, books, or articles recommend, is a risky undertaking for any of us. It shouldn't be done without medical consultation. Laura's diet was irrationally conceived and dangerous to her health. The self-induced vomiting was a panicky measure, designed to hasten weight loss and based on the wild notion that once food was in the mouth it yielded its nutritional value to the body and then could be discarded. Laura's chances of remaining thin, even if she had avoided the complication of pneumonia, were quite poor. Her dieting had been motivated largely by desperation. When we are past the crisis situation that compelled us to lessen our food intake, the urge to become thin also lessens.

Undereating and dangerous malnutrition occur in a peculiar condition known as *anorexia nervosa,* where weight loss because of insufficient food intake can become life-threatening. It usually occurs in young girls, accompanied by absence of menstrual periods (amenorrhea). It is not a common disorder, but emotional upset plays a major role in it and psychological clues signal its development. These include an underlying depression as manifested in peculiar attitudes toward eating and food. There are also many rationalizations about the need to be thin, and a denial that anything is wrong. A plump mother may be in the background, or one who has made eating a big issue in the past. There is ignorance or abnormal thinking about sex and pregnancy, with biting, chewing, swallowing prominent in the fantasies about them. Preventive psychotherapy is essential, because once *anorexia nervosa* becomes established, the outlook is less favorable. In more severe cases hospitalization, intravenous feeding, and even more stringent physical measures are required in addition to continuous emotional support. And all these measures may at times fail, and then death from starvation and its complications occurs.

An increasing number of teen-agers and young adults from nonpoor families eat inadequately. Drugs may blunt their appetite or result in their lack of attention to proper food intake. Some of these youngsters stick to diets which promise miraculous benefits for mind or body but deprive them of essential nutrients. It may seem strange that people who are bright and informed about many things show an extraordinary gullibility or naiveté regarding diet and personal hygiene. But the explanation can often be found in the individual's emotional hangups, which are related to rebellious, attention-gaining, ascetic, or self-destructive needs. These are all signs that reason will be overcome at times. Their prominent presence is a warning that sickness may not be far away.

EMOTION, NUTRITION—AND SPORTS

Although all the psychological factors we've been discussing are no secret in the scientific world, some nutrition experts still pay little attention to their value in predicting health disturbances associated with weight loss or gain, or eating problems in general. I heard one authority exchange opinions with a famous pitcher about how athletes keep in condition. They got to talking about what happens to pitchers during crucial games. The pitcher mentioned the six or eight pounds he tended to lose because of great stress during each close game. The expert, paying no attention, launched into a discussion of excessive perspiration because of warm weather, loss of vitamins, minerals, and other micro-nutrients, muscle fatigue, leg cramps. Not one single word about emotions: the stress of competition, the need to make or maintain a place on the team, the impact of crowd noises, the carryover of tensions from other sources, the anxiety which could interfere with coordination, tighten muscles, blunt acquired skills or upset metabolism, increase water loss, and enhance fatigue. Yet the pitcher himself, with no scientific background, had intuitively put his finger on what was probably the most important factor—the triggering effect of emotion on all these physical processes.

Many of us, similarly, have an intuitive feeling that our emotions are somehow tied in with our eating habits, even though our own problems may not be as severe as some of the cases we have just read about. We know we pick at our food when we are angry—or perhaps can't even swallow at all if we are in deep distress. We know a given food can taste better when we are happy than when we are sad. We know we tend to indulge ourselves in an extra beer or martini, potato chips, peanuts, or a too-fattening dessert when we feel disappointed and left out of things. And maybe quite a bit of this is normal and good for us; it's a kind of outlet for tensions which otherwise might build up in us. It's a way of patting ourselves on the back and giving ourselves a lift, which we sometimes deserve.

But what if you feel that things are getting out of hand? Hopefully you will feel motivated to get medical advice that also takes your emotions into consideration. It doesn't have to be a specialized, deep exploration of your unconscious, or prolonged, high-priced therapy. Maybe giving yourself time to think about yourself, or talking openly with someone you trust, will give you a better incentive than just appealing to your willpower—which often doesn't work, so that you later feet more guilty than ever.

For those of us who are parents, the people we've discussed in this chapter have a double significance—for ourselves and for our children. Let's not blind ourselves to indications that an eating problem is in the making for them. Look for signs of emotional deprivation in the child, for indications that eating is serving as a substitute for affection, that there is an overemphasis on the importance of food, that there is identification with parental figures who are obese or who have unusual eating habits themselves, that there is a rebellious attitude to food. Expert psychological advice can help us help our children avoid faulty eating habits leading to obesity or malnutrition later in life, when treatment is much more difficult. An ounce of foresight prevents many nervous pounds of flesh.

13

Will You Get Sick on Vacation?

Writers of travel books tell their readers to get as many facts as they can about the places they're going to visit and to plan their trip with care. Good advice. They go on to warn that a sour disposition will spoil it all. Useful warning. Then come more directions: think of the trip as not so complicated, and the nervousness about visiting new or unknown places will disappear. Maybe. Or, they say: forget your problems. If you can.

Many of us know in a superficial way that tension can make a vacation unpleasant. And many of us are also familiar with the suggestions and reassurances—as well as the encouragement to use denial in dealing with any nervous strain before we start out on a trip. However, few of us are aware that emotional clues can alert us to the possibility of physical sickness on vacation. Hitherto, most explanations for such disorders have focused entirely on physical aspects such as unsanitary conditions, strange foods, different water, lack of immunity to new germs. The emphasis, moreover, has been on the infectious illnesses. But travelers may suffer from many noncontagious disorders. Can these, and even germ-caused disease, be anticipated by psychological indicators? Yes, the clues that have been discussed in previous chapters are useful in predicting whether we'll be vulnerable to *any* physical illness during our holiday.

EMOTIONS DON'T TAKE A HOLIDAY

First, we can review in our minds whether we already are under a great strain, even before we take off. Will the albatross of internal emotional conflict accompany us no matter how far we go? Are we trying to forget, or to escape from our problems? How? By retreating to a place free of tensions, where we'll be pampered, where we can comfortably regress in the service of being reconstituted emotionally? Or are we going to be rushing around frenetically, trying to be diverted by new stimuli, crowds, turmoil? Retreat may soothe, overactivity may aggravate tensions. But not always. So how much inactivity and how much diversion? That's difficult to answer without knowing the specifics of each person's needs. To a certain extent, new places, languages, sights, sounds, eating and drinking customs, climate, and time changes will be stressful. Then it's a matter of how we adapt to the unfamiliar. Do we take it in stride—even thrive on it, as some seem to do—or get tense or respond with a body disorder? We have already acquired some wisdom about this; we know something about how we react under stress. If we gave it more thought, we could form some opinion of how we'll do on our vacation, instead of proceeding blindly.

But let's continue with our self-appraisal. Is suffering a way of life with us—whether at work or on vacation—so we can *never* enjoy anything? Some people never take time off from their work. Others do, but are thoroughly uncomfortable every minute they're away; work is the only way they can avoid their emotional difficulties, and such a pattern, once it's set, becomes difficult to change. On the other hand, some people far removed from their familiar surroundings are able to act out impulses they would ordinarily suppress. Another question to consider is this: Though we're going on vacation or actually are on vacation, are we preoccupied

141

with thoughts of someone close to us who's ill or has recently been ill? Are we repeatedly dreaming of physical disorder? Have we become careless—overexerting ourselves, eating and drinking injudiciously, not getting enough sleep, becoming involved in dangerous adventures? These are signs that our bodies will suffer.

New stimuli on our vacation may distract us from our troubles. But as we have noted, they may also produce tension. A critical question is whether psychological outlets for such tension have been shut off or have become insufficient. Have we stopped being irritated, stopped blaming others? Do we get no satisfaction out of sightseeing or shopping in new places? Do we feel dull, uninterested, even apathetic? All these are indications that physical illness is likely, even though we're on a holiday.

For anyone who has a chronic illness and is planning a vacation, all the factors set forth above may have a bearing on the possibility of recurrence and/or aggravation of the condition.

Sometimes illness comes late—as the vacation is ending and we return to the familiar. Anticipation, new stimuli, healthy excitement, preoccupation with details of planning as we begin our travels, may counteract or at least mask any untoward emotional reactions. On our return to the familiar, to the old unresolved problems, to the rat race, our conflicts may intensify and often there may be a letdown. This can range from slight to severe, and it may be accompanied or replaced by physical disturbances.

HIGH FLIER

Let us now consider some examples. Ilsa was the department store's prettiest, youngest, brightest buyer. It was vacation time for her, but she was planning to combine it with some quiet business, a coup for the store and for herself.

The store would get an exclusive on some Japanese goods, and she might be made head buyer. She called it quiet business, but in fact it involved a deliberate attempt to oust her boss, a veteran of many years with the firm but reluctant to retire. There was another slight flaw in what on the surface seemed like a well-planned vacation. Her doctor had noted that her blood pressure was a little high. He thought the tensions of her job might be bringing it up. So he agreed that the distractions and pleasures of a trip to the Orient would be just the right thing, in addition to the medicine he was prescribing. What he did not realize was that she was planning to take her job tensions right along on the trip—that she could not take a vacation from her need to be number one.

All her life, despite her many talents, Ilsa had been plagued by feelings of inferiority. Is it possible to feel inferior even if you are an attractive person everyone *else* thinks is a success? Yes, some people cover up an unrelenting sense of inadequacy by an extreme drive to get ahead. That's what Ilsa did. She wanted to beat everybody. *Everybody.* When she was a little girl she wanted to impress the big people in her life, but they seemed indifferent to her childish triumphs and accomplishments. She never got over that. Now, when she herself was grown up, no matter how much success she had, deep down she still felt small and had to prove herself over and over again. These unresolved issues had not erupted from behind the barriers that had been erected against them. Ilsa had not felt anxious, angry, guilty, or upset in any way, nor did she now as she began her vacation. This very absence of any noticeable emotional reaction was an indication that her trip might not be without unpleasant consequences.

Ilsa left the doctor's office with a prescription but forgot to get it filled. There were so many details to take care of before the trip. She remembered the prescription again only when she was on the plane and had a bad headache.

A couple of aspirins quickly took care of that; but while she had relaxed very quickly on other vacations a few hours after she had left the big city, this time she remained keyed up. It was a change that she tried to ignore.

In certain respects, except for the unexpected nervousness and headaches, which kept recurring, the trip seemed a success. She got the account, and on her return, top management moved her into the head buyer's position. It was with expectant triumph that Ilsa phoned her mother, her doubting mother who had always belittled her. But all she got was a slurred "That's nice, dear." (Her mother had taken to drinking.) Ilsa felt let down, then strangely apathetic. She began to have unpleasant dreams of plane crashes in which many people were killed. Then came an unexpected and unwelcome bonus—the nagging headaches got worse. Some weeks later, when they didn't go away, she became alarmed and ran to her doctor again. He shook his head after he checked her blood pressure: "Two hundred over one hundred. Too high." This time she was uncomfortable enough to pay attention. This time she did not forget to have the prescription filled.

She thought back to her vacation and had some glimmerings that it had not been a true rest because—though her surroundings had been different—she had continued to be driven by the same old need to get ahead. Her competitive fury had been bottled up. Her successes had not resolved her emotional conflicts, had not provided a satisfactory outlet for them. Things became even worse after she had done her boss out of a job and had repressed her fury at her uncaring, alcoholic mother. Feelings of rage and guilt were piling up in her. Now she had the added burden of proving herself able to cope with her new responsibilities. A warning voice within her told her it was time to cool her emotions or suffer even higher blood pressure and its consequences. But not all of us learn such a valuable lesson.

ANGER—AND THEN THERE WAS ONE

Mr. and Mrs. Dispew were trying hard to relax and enjoy their trip, but they took along on vacation their incompatibility of many years. Mrs. Dispew was letting her husband have it for the thousandth time, criticizing his table manners as they were having dinner in a topnotch French restaurant in a lovely garden setting. An expensive place, but it was their big splurge. Mrs. Dispew was anxious, more than usual. She had put on her best clothes for this special occasion but felt uneasy in the presence of the smartly dressed men and women who all seemed to be rich, urbane, even aristocratic. So she could enjoy nothing, neither the beautiful garden, the delicious food, nor the faultless service. And she would not let her husband enjoy any of it. The cocktails had made her voice strident. "Get your elbows off the table," she kept telling him. "If you had any manners at all, you'd know better than to sit with your elbows on the table." Her husband, who never argued with her, tried to joke about her complaints, but she would have none of his humor. He protested that his elbows *were* off the table, and for a few moments there was an uneasy silence as they toyed with their food.

Then the habit of a lifetime reasserted itself, and one of Mr. Dispew's elbows returned to its resting place on the table. His wife renewed her attack. By this time Mr. Dispew had become desperately self-conscious. Instead of two elbows he seemed to have twenty. His own tension had risen so sharply that he felt confused. His wife's eyes were darting around the patio. Had anyone noticed her husband's bad manners? The familiar symptoms of indigestion began to affect Mr. Dispew—he hardly touched his dessert. His wife finally shut up in the cab on the way back to the hotel.

Dispew was silent. He was thinking how, back home after an argument, especially when those chest pains would bother him, he would usually get away from his wife by going down to the Brown Jug for a few slow beers and a friendly cussing session with the boys. By the time he got home he would have worked off his anger and his wife would be asleep. But here in this unfamiliar place, where could he go, what could he do? His indigestion got worse; the oppressive feeling spread to his chest. He could not express any anger toward his wife. Instead he felt like a boiler about to burst under tremendous pressure. And no safety valve. All these were signs of impending trouble, and all, unfortunately, went unheeded. In the hotel room Mrs. Dispew renewed her attack—"Elbow—table—elbow—table"—until he fled, on the pretext of getting something for his "heartburn." But the powder he took in the hotel pharmacy didn't make him feel any better. He decided to take a walk. The night air was cool, and there was a bit of wind, but he was burning up. Dispew had never felt like this before. The pain in his chest, the tension—so great he could feel it in his neck and face muscles. The pain began to go down his left arm; his elbow was aching. A policeman stared at him as he walked by unsteadily. A girl asked him if he was looking for a good time. On he went . . . .

Mrs. Dispew, who had fallen asleep still muttering about the disgrace her husband had brought on them, was wakened by a telephone call from the police. The inquest showed that Mr. Dispew had dropped dead of coronary thrombosis, acute, massive, while walking the streets shortly before midnight. It did not reveal that Mr. Dispew finally had reached the limit of tolerance of his long pent-up fury at his wife. That repressed rage that he had avoided facing for so many years had finally caught up with him, thousands of miles away from home, in a place where he could not relieve it or his heart pains by running off and joining the fellows. And its immense energies struck his body with full force.

For Mrs. Dispew, the need to make a nice impression—so easy to do back home—had run into trouble in the frighteningly fancy restaurant. But tension already had been building in them both, chiefly because they had chosen to spend their vacation in a setting so totally unfamiliar to them that neither was comfortable. Maybe the tragedy—though not the basic incompatibility, of course—might have been averted or delayed if they had chosen a less pretentious restaurant (where elbows wouldn't have been such a big issue) or a less pretentious hotel (near a neighborhood bistro that might have been as homey as Mr. Dispew's bar). If only they had heeded the warning signs!

Many of us make this sort of mistake on our vacation; we try to fulfill dreams of living like the jet set, like royalty. Such make-believe may act as a safety valve for tensions as long as we can handle it and recognize its limited usefulness. All too often, however, like the Dispews, we blindly choose places where we can't unwind, and thus we make ourselves doubly miserable. Then, if we know from past experience that nervous strain causes our bodies to act up, we are risking the possibility of a severe physical reaction. So it behooves us, when making vacation plans, to examine our hangups, unrealistic wishes, and body reactivity—indicators of possible trouble—and to choose holiday sites that will bring true relaxation.

NO ESCAPE

Though it is hard to leave our emotional troubles behind when we travel, there are people who succeed in doing this. Some people can forget for a good part of the trip. Some can really escape, not only from difficulties such as an unpleasant home or a hated job, but even from their consciences. It is not unknown for a frustrated woman and man—married or unmarried—liberated by distance, by being in a setting where they cannot be questioned by family or friends, to have the affair of a lifetime. But most of us can't forget at all, no matter how great the distraction of travel or the separation from those who know us.

Consider what happened to Max, widower, and Mary, unattached—both seeking escape. He was fleeing from the pressure and routine of the garment business and the incessant demands of his relatives; she, from a spinster's boredom and no family at all. They were a study in contrasts: he was a depressed, heavyset fifty-five; she had a perpetual smile, was slender and thirtyish. He was complaining as was his custom, and she was trying to be cheerful—at least he was paying the bills. But he had a bad sore throat. Something real to gripe about. He had not had a cold the whole winter, when he had been driving himself through those long hours at the office. It was then that he conceived the idea of having his first fling abroad—with a sophisticate's touch of indulging in a mistress.

But Max couldn't enjoy it. Ever since his wife had died, five years before, he had dreamed of living it up and having fun. But this idea seemed as immoral as his married life had been conventional. Same place in the mountains year after year for vacation. No fun or sex. Nothing but his business. He had to stifle the idea, which arose from time to time, that he was even a little bit relieved that his wife had died. After her death his business became all the more his whole life, except that sometimes he had a secret dream of being a sexual hero, and then he masturbated. But he kept telling himself he really had to do something about women, before it was too late. And Mary was so agreeable, so accommodating. If only he didn't react with such guilt. If only he could get rid of that memory of his wife whenever he wanted to enjoy himself. Maybe distance from his familiar surroundings would do it. Maybe he would even marry again, if Mary would have him.

But though his reasoning made it seem easy, his conscience wouldn't buy it. Underneath he had to atone for trying to get a little pleasure, because he felt he wasn't supposed to. His lot in life was to suffer and to be wretched; his conscience was that severe and irrational: "Don't step out of line, don't do anything that convention forbids, don't masturbate, don't have an affair, don't have any fun." The experiences of childhood had lingered on: the stern parents, forbidding and punitive. After any little thing that wasn't just right, he would feel the lash of the strap or the scorn of the bitter words. And that was the way he treated himself, though somewhere in him was rebellion. In fact, he thought his guilty feelings had disappeared as he started on his adventure, but recollections of his wife's illness—her "double" pneumonia—began to harass him by day, and dreams of choking haunted him by night. Then he got sick. It was to be his punishment, lay him up with a fever for three days, and leave him with a hacking cough for the rest of the trip. A hacking cough all through Spain and Italy, which took most of the joy out of his affair. And then Mary caught his cold. She also was atoning. Despite her cheerful appearance, the little gremlins of guilt were secretly bothering her too. She knew that she really didn't like Max. She was only going along for the ride. Getting a cold made her feel more virtuous about being kept.

The vacation didn't turn out as either one had dreamed it—a chance to break loose from the old, established ways and be uninhibited for once in their lives. But the indications of trouble had been there from the beginning, especially the need to suffer one way or another. Unfortunately Mary and Max had been unaware of these signs.

When many of us make vacation plans, we expect, unrealistically, that a change of scene and a couple of weeks away from the rat race are going to cure the deep tensions we have been unable or unwilling to face the rest of the year. We may get some relief. But a cure? That's something else again.

WHEN TRAVEL ISN'T THE ANSWER

Similarly, many lonely people yearn for a change in their monotonous lives and dream of being with their loved ones who may be in faraway places. To be with them and savor the excitement of travel—that would seem to be a double pleasure. But not always. Mrs. Gresham was a sad-looking woman in her mid-sixties. She had what she called Nassau tummy, but if you've traveled, you know the same malady confronts the tourist wherever he goes, although under a different name in different places. There's Montezuma's revenge in Mexico, Tokyo toots in the Orient, or the Italian trots. You'll hear travelers complain that they get it in your own hometown, though people in town don't seem to get it until *they* travel somewhere else.

So was Mrs. Gresham suffering from something called Nassau tummy, or was she suffering from emotion she couldn't name, couldn't release, but which was upsetting her body? The bags under her eyes swelled and her face appeared even more forlorn as she spoke: "Imagine, just twelve hours before, I was sitting in my London house, not knowing what to do with myself. I'm three times a widow, and the loneliness gets to be intolerable. Then my son phoned. So unexpected after six months. Next week he's going on to America, and I probably won't see him for another year. He's my one and only. It's not easy being alone back home. You're not wanted by the other couples. As for those widow clubs and stuff—that's not for me. Not a line, not a word from my son for six months, then this call, inviting me for a holiday down in Nassau. I got so excited. But the moment I checked into the hotel, I started to vomit. My son's been so busy I've hardly had a chance to talk with him since I got here. I was so sick. Not just vomiting, but diarrhea too. All that good food, and I couldn't touch any of it. I don't know if it was a bug or that water."

The hotel water? Perfectly safe. New intestinal bugs?

Maybe, but hardly likely, because the symptoms began so soon. Tension? Plenty. Listen further to Mrs. Gresham: "I have a great need to be with people. The big question for me has been what to do about my loneliness. Well, at least my daffodils will be coming out when I get back home. And there'll be the familiar faces of the neighborhood. Right now I've found a lover here in Nassau." (Long pause.) "Seven years old and such a sweet child."

Mrs. Gresham had a great deal of trouble indeed adapting to her loneliness. She looked for easy solutions—especially from other people—but had few, if any, resources of inner security to fall back on when the going got really rough. Yet she rarely acknowledged, rarely was aware of, her extreme chronic bitterness. What did it all add up to? Because she was unable to find a satisfactory solution to her problems, her body bore the brunt of her unexpressed feelings. That had been so all her life. Now, that anger Mrs. Gresham felt toward her son exploded in vomiting and diarrhea. This history of body reactions to stress, of pent-up rage which was repeatedly denied, indicated that what seemed like a fun trip would turn out to be the opposite. How much better it would have been for her if she had gained some insight into her problems before she embarked on the trip. In her situation, professional help was needed.

Reading guidebooks, calling travel agents, or booking into the very best hotels is not enough to ensure a great vacation. Neither are the sage precautions about jet lag or disturbance in our circadian rhythms. We also need to review our emotional makeup for indications of possible physical disturbance while we're on a trip. A crucial factor in a happy holiday is asking ourselves what we really want from it—rest, fun, a change of pace, new sights and sounds, a magic solution to our problems, escape from our troubles—and whether just the vacation itself is going to do the trick.

14

When to Expect Sexual Disorders

Most people know in a general way that sexual hangups are related to disturbed emotions, that the basis for this relationship is set early in life, and that the conflicts may remain dormant, only to be activated by later stress. Perhaps less well known is the fact that once these disorders become established, they are hard to treat. This is true, for example, of impotence, lack of sexual response in women, and menstrual difficulties that don't respond to hormones. Doctors are confronted daily by puzzling problems involving infertility, the use and effectiveness of contraceptives, and complications following sterilization. Obviously, anticipating these conditions would spare many people untold suffering and expense. Recently, specific clues have been studied which can predict the likelihood of bodily disturbances associated with sexuality in the adult before they actually develop.

WARNING SIGNALS

What are these indications?

(1) Activation of: (a) long-standing latent concerns over virility or feminine appeal; (b) old misconceptions about sex, picturing it as dirty, brutal, forbidden, debilitating, controlling, etc.; (c) strongly feminine impulses in men and strongly masculine impulses in women which lead to conflict over sexual identity. These

are derived partly from disturbances in identification with significant family figures or current surrogates.

(2) An increase in self-centeredness—narcissism—which tends to exclude genuine interest in the sexual partner.

(3) Intensified denial of troublesome thoughts, feelings, or behavior.

(4) Relative blocking of psychological outlets for sexual conflicts.

(5) Awareness of guilt over sexuality, followed by a rapid disappearance of these feelings.

(6) Pent-up irritability for all kinds of reasons, but particularly related to frustration of infantile sexual impulses.

(7) Dreams full of sexual symbols and characterized by anxiety to the point of disturbing sleep.

PORTENTS OF IMPOTENCE

Let's start with the case of Tom, a self-educated auto worker, who had had many brief affairs with women at the plant where he was employed. But when he became involved with a debutante (they had met at a peace demonstration) and after she told him of her father's violent opposition to the relationship, Tom had twinges of insecurity. For the first time in years, he began to have doubts about his masculinity—the first sign of trouble—followed by occasional difficulty in maintaining an erection. In the past, especially after some setback at work, when he had temporarily lost confidence in himself, he could usually quell his uneasiness by fantasies of being able to seduce all women. Now this didn't work. Actually he had not resolved his childhood confusion about his sexual identity. He was the youngest and only boy in a family of five children. His father, a traveling salesman, was rarely home. Tom was turned into a sissy by his mother and sisters. Later he tried to overcome this by acting like a Don Juan.

Tom married his debutante. He insisted they not have

children for a while, but she quickly became pregnant. She had a difficult time, being bothered for months by nausea and vomiting. It was then that Tom noticed he was preoccupied with sexual fantasies he had not had since childhood, when he had often pictured himself as a girl. This, together with secret preliminary nipple and anal self-stimulation, now aroused him to masturbate, but he avoided sexual relations with his wife, using the excuse that she was sick (though she wasn't *that* sick). On several occasions he had nightmares that *he* was pregnant and had a miscarriage. Then a new worry stuck in his mind—that something might happen to his wife or baby. Actually it was a way of concealing his hostility to them—to his wife for turning her attention to the pregnancy, and toward the baby for displacing him in his wife's affections. He felt very guilty about his growing disinterest in his wife, and then suddenly that stopped bothering him. In fact, all his troublesome thoughts and feelings seemed to subside. All these signs pointed to some physical disturbance. And, indeed, when his wife began feeling better and he tried again to have intercourse with her, he found himself repeatedly impotent. But that wasn't the end of it. A month before his wife was due to deliver, he developed nausea, lost his appetite, and tired easily. One toothache after another plagued him. He took to bed but refused to see either his physician or his dentist. A week later his wife delivered a seven-pound healthy baby boy, whereupon Tom immediately felt fit enough to get up and hand out cigars. His symptoms rapidly disappeared, except for his impotence.

What had been wrong with Tom? The doctor who subsequently gave him his annual checkup at the union clinic made one diagnosis: Couvade syndrome. Few people have heard of it, yet there is good reason to believe it occurs far more often than we can actually prove. This is because the husband is unaware of the emotional signals that precede its development and doesn't let anyone know about his strange symptoms, or else because his illness is attributed to a virus. However, surveys indicate that at least ten percent and perhaps as many as fifty percent of all expectant fathers suffer from symptoms that mimic the discomforts of pregnancy. There have even been instances reported in which the pregnant woman's *father* became sick! Interestingly, most wives questioned seemed unaware of some relationship between their pregnancy and their husband's illness.

But what about Tom's impotence? He had not revealed that or his sexual practices and associated fantasies to the doctor. And all too often, at the beginning of a serious illness or before an operation, signs of a patient's activated concern about virility are missed, because he doesn't talk about it and his physician doesn't ask. Later, the patient becomes impotent while the doctor is busy looking for physical causes which usually are not the answer. If the patient's psychological state had been as carefully explored as his physical condition, the doctor would have been alerted to the likelihood that impotence would develop, and preventive psychological measures could have been instituted.

Let us consider another case of impotence. One of my patients, Eddy, a single man in his late twenties, had been very friendly for years with a married couple his own age. After the husband was killed in an accident, Eddy continued to see the widow. They became more intimate physically, but though she wanted to have intercourse, he held back. His uneasiness and reserve were signals of underlying anxiety and guilt over erotic thoughts he had had about her while her husband was still alive. He also worried about his virility and whether he would be able to match her late husband's sexual achievements (of which he actually knew nothing).

When these thoughts and feelings disappeared, though without being resolved, they were replaced by vivid fantasies—long forgotten—about his mother. She had played upon his erotic interests by acting seductively. Sometimes she would plop herself face down on a bed, pull up her nightgown, and ask him to sprinkle some powder on a painful pimple on her buttocks. Yet, if he showed any sign of being excited, it would be quickly squelched by feelings of embarrassment and fear of what his alcoholic, brutish father might do if he found out about these intimate scenes. It was even more perplexing to overhear his mother tell a woman neighbor about his being a "cute little doctor" and their both laughing about it.

Another memory returned: When he was six, his favorite aunt came to stay for a while at Eddy's home and slept in a spare bed in his bedroom. Once, when she came in late, he awoke and silently watched her undress. The sight of her stark naked body excited him. Another night, as she took off her underpants, some blood leaked out between her legs and she hurriedly went into the bathroom. Eddy was so frightened by this he never looked again during his aunt's short stay. Because he felt that sexual thoughts were bad and punishable, he quickly pushed them out of his awareness, and there they remained repressed until his adolescence. It was then that his aunt suddenly reappeared as a central figure in his masturbation fantasies, with his uncle always absent.

Eddy had ignored these recollections, not realizing that their incestuous nature was making him guilt ridden and could lead to impotence in actual sexual relations with women.

There are other signs that impotence may develop. One of these is *over*concern for the woman. The man begins to be afraid that he will hurt his sexual partner if intercourse takes place. However, here the anxiety may be a cover for *hidden* hostile impulses toward the woman. Another signal of impotence is a fear of losing semen. Strange as it may seem, some men have a neurotic belief that semen is a vital substance whose emission weakens the body. Usually men with this notion were frightened in childhood or adolescence by reading or being told the myth that masturbation weakens the body. Similar groundless fear is found in men who were misinformed earlier in life that semen was a dirty substance; this fear may be a sign that there will be difficulty with ejaculation.

Severe impotence, once established, is difficult to treat. So familiarity with early warning signals (usually psychological) is important in order to be able to prevent it or lessen its severity. If these signals are heeded, treatment focusing on relief of tensions, airing of problems, especially those of a sexual nature, correction of false beliefs about sex, and information about proper love techniques may be sufficient to prevent the condition. In cases where impotence has become established and is severe, hypnosis, conditioning treatment, and different forms of psychotherapy have all been used with variable success.

FORECAST: PREMATURE EJACULATION

Another male sexual disorder whose development can be foretold is *ejaculatio praecox* or premature ejaculation. It occurs occasionally in most men, especially if they have developed concern about their virility (even though they may be unaware of this feeling) at the beginning of their erotic experiences with women or after periods of abstinence. The primary indications that it may be more than a transient experience are a focusing on forepleasure satisfactions and a deep-seated but repressed hostility toward women. This emotion will already have been expressed in disguised fashion and in many nonsexual ways, particularly in everyday attitudes and behavior. At some point which cannot be exactly determined but corresponds to a critical buildup of negative feelings, these may then interfere with the sexual act. Ejaculation is triggered almost at the moment the vagina is entered or very shortly thereafter, usually before the woman has had a chance to reach orgasm herself, leaving her unsatisfied and upset.

A number of men who consulted me because of premature ejaculation had particular trouble in being aware of, and in expressing, anger. They were married to women who were highly critical of them. Usually the patients' reaction was to work like crazy to be successful, and they took some of their hostility out in their business affairs. However, plenty was left over for their wives, and it was expressed in the form of premature ejaculation. It was useful for these men to become more aware of their anger, how they were expressing it, and why. But once the condition is established, when it is repetitious and unremitting, it is difficult to treat, no matter what approach is used.

IS "FRIGIDITY" PREDICTABLE?

In women, lack of sexual arousal (still commonly known as frigidity), together with insufficient or absent vaginal lubrication, is a disturbance even more common than impotence in men. However, women can engage in sexual intercourse whether they are interested or not. A woman also can conceive without being sexually aroused; so women can conceal their lack of arousal from others, and even from themselves.

General lack of interest in sex, feelings of disgust at the very thought of it, unpleasant bodily sensations during physical intimacy, fears of being hurt or taken advantage of—all are warnings that sexual relations will not lead to pleasant feelings or orgasm. The anxiety is often due to the persistence of childhood misconceptions about sex, picturing it as sadomasochistic, dirty, and forbidden. Some women are preoccupied by differences in male and female genitalia. They want, consciously or unconsciously, to get what men have, just as some men envy female physique and ability to bear children. Such women can become so hostile and upset during intercourse—to the point of feeling themselves abused or wanting to deprive men of their masculinity—that they have no sexual sensation. Psychological conflicts involving strong emotional attachments to other women may be a more subtle and less commonly recognized cause of lack of sexual response to men. And, until recently, the double standard exerted a powerful cultural deterrent to sexual response in women.

Again, it's better to take preventive measures against this condition than to deal with it after it has become established, because then treatment is less apt to be successful. And many approaches have been tried: reassurance, explanation (often with both partners present), intensive individual psychotherapy, instruction about proper lubrication and gradual penetration of the vagina, deconditioning procedures, and individual interviews with a therapist, plus separate "special instruction" in sexual technique by an "experienced partner." With none of these approaches is the outcome certain.

CURSE OF THE "CURSE"

Menstruation often has been referred to as "the curse" or other equally ugly names, but nowadays it appears to be less burdensome. New medication to prevent fluid retention and pain, use of modern contraceptives, and an increasing sense of liberation and equality—with their psychological effects—all play a role in lessening bodily discomfort from menstruation. Hitherto, a considerable emphasis has been put on the role hormones play during menstruation, so much so that emotional conflicts present since childhood are not considered by some doctors as having any influence on this process. This is an extreme point of view which leaves out important data. Actually, my studies show that late, skipped, irregular, painful, scanty, or hemorrhagic periods may be anticipated when there is a psychological history of the following: (1) old and new antagonisms between yourself and mother (or mother-surrogates); (2) an increase in your dependency on her or in competitive feelings toward her; (3) feelings of being rejected by a father who favored males; (4) long-standing ambivalence about being a woman, especially if there is strong identification with a suffering, gynecologically sick mother; (5) unusual preoccupation with details about the menstrual cycle; (6) recent problems at work, with children, husband, or boyfriend, or lack of male companionship. The more of these factors that are present, the more likely the menstrual problem. But, as with the other ailments we have discussed, the most significant indicator of impending menstrual difficulties is the relative absence of psychological response to whatever is upsetting you.

A patient of mine, a career woman holding a junior executive position in a bank, talked a great deal about competing with the men there. But when she was passed up for a promotion—which went to a male colleague who was more qualified—she seemed unaffected. Her lack of emotional response was a sign that her feelings could be having an impact on her body. By her activity, the patient had always tried to deny being identified with her frail and anemic-looking mother—a kitchen slave—who was constantly tired. Recently the mother had had her uterus removed because her doctor had found a suspicious mass there. The patient wondered whether she would become ill in the same way and then not be able to have any children. The strong, though resisted identification with her mother was a further sign that her reproductive system might bear the brunt of her tensions. Shortly thereafter, she noted increasingly painful, irregular periods.

In her own words: "I wonder about my irregularity.

Besides, I also get constipated when I get the curse. I have trouble with Tampax and it doesn't protect me. During my last period I was standing on our favorite Oriental rug and started to leak. Afterward I had pain with intercourse and even with orgasm, which I never had before. Maybe my womb's dropping down or tipping. Maybe a cancer is growing there."

The need for a gynecological examination was discussed. It was quickly arranged and revealed several fibroids that had not been noted before. They were the cause of the difficult periods. Watchful waiting, but no immediate surgery, was advised by the gynecologist.

DO I OR DON'T I?

While some women are relieved by the occurrence of menstruation as the monthly reminder that they are not pregnant, others who very much want to get pregnant become depressed. The thought "I want a baby and I'm going to have one" can become a steady drumbeat in a woman's brain. Especially when she is not fertile and has a great need to prove she *can* conceive—perhaps to rescue a failing marriage or to hold her husband's affection. Such intense longing signals that strange things may happen to her body and she may develop pseudocyesis, a condition simulating pregnancy.

But the thought "I *don't* want a baby" can become just as impelling a force in a woman's mind, though not in her awareness, when she *is* pregnant. Often such a negative attitude—stirred up by fears of being a terrible mother, or not wanting to be burdened by children, or by her husband's disinterest and neglect—persistent though it may be, tends to be obscured. In fact, the woman may protest (too much, since it is an attempt to conceal the opposite) how concerned she is about the pregnancy going well, especially when spotting, staining, and outright bleeding occur. This extreme and deceptive emotional reaction may forecast an unpleasant physical development. The powerful rejection of the baby mentally reaches a dramatic climax when the woman miscarries.

Though emotional conflicts about having a baby affect a woman's physiology, few doctors know how to investigate these at the same time the pregnancy is confirmed, and so they miss the indications those conflicts provide of possible future trouble.

ANTICIPATING INFERTILITY

Infertility is distressing and puzzling to a couple who "say" they want children, especially when all physical factors have been considered and treated. How often then do they or their physician think of the disturbed emotions which warn of this? Where do you look for these signs?

Frequently they are concealed in the interaction of the husband and wife, in the emotional effect they have on each other. Incompatibility, unremitting hostility, individual and collective hangups about sex, camouflaged lack of desire for children, selfish, infantile attitudes which make the husband want to be taken care of—without rivals—by the wife (or vice versa), or unrealistic overemphasis on independence—all are indicators of a troubled relationship. In their presence, interference with normal reproductive functions becomes likely when psychological release—by daydreaming, quarreling, acting out with other sexual partners, separation, etc.—is insufficient to relieve the accumulated tensions. The following is an example: A patient of mine, a learned researcher in his prime, had been married for five years to a career woman. The couple wanted children (at least they thought so), and when their initial efforts failed, each had a thorough checkup, that is, a physical one. Hers was negative. His revealed a low sperm count probably due to an old inflammation of the testicles occurring as a complication of mumps during adolescence. They were advised to adopt a child. But the wife actually was more interested in her career than in children; it was the husband who really wanted a child. They didn't take any steps toward adoption and finally abandoned the idea.

The marriage began to deteriorate as their personalities and aspirations clashed more and more. The wife did not enjoy sexual intercourse, and after the checkups blamed her lack of enthusiasm on her husband's "sterility." Meanwhile he tried to overcompensate for his stirred-up inferiority feelings by being sexually vigorous and was increasingly frustrated because of her unresponsiveness. All these were additional signs that emotional factors were strongly involved in their infertility problem. Their arguments became so bitter that they decided to live apart.

It was at this point that the husband entered treatment, feeling dejected and a failure as a man, despite his oustanding academic reputation. With therapy, his confidence in himself gradually increased; he also became more aware of his current extreme rage and its earlier roots involving his domineering mother. His wife filed for divorce, but he weathered this stress and, in fact, became involved with a younger woman. One day, shortly before the divorce decree became final, his mistress joyously told him she was pregnant. And it was actually so. Under favorable emotional conditions, with development of a true love relationship, and fully satisfying sexual release, his sterility had become an outdated label. This is not to deny that infertility has physical aspects, but these don't necessarily tell the whole story. Psychological signs may point to trouble conceiving, if they are looked for (and understood) early, when a couple is planning to have children. Then treatment can be *both* psychological and physical.

PREDICTION OF TROUBLE WITH CONTRACEPTION

In the opposite situation to pregnancy, birth control, it is also true that specific psychological clues can help predict problems in the use and effectiveness of contraceptives.

A couple's attitude toward birth control is not always what it seems to be. Take the case of Mrs. Smith, mother of two. She has come to the birth control clinic because ostensibly she doesn't want any more children at this time. She has a brief talk with the doctor which, unfortunately, skips over her marital problems and sexual needs, her adaptive responses and defenses, the availability (or lack) of psychological outlets, activity of her conscience—all indicators of possible trouble with contraception. Then she is given a prescription for the pill. After taking it for a while, Mrs. Smith becomes depressed and uninterested in sex. She stops taking the pill. Then she's no longer depressed. In this instance experts would claim the depression was due to hormones in the pill.

But another woman, Mrs. Jones, also after a similarly perfunctory interview, is fitted for an intrauterine device (IUD), which is a plastic coil or loop inserted into the uterus, which some women cannot tolerate. They may bleed or experience cramps. Sometimes they expel it. In Mrs. Jones's case, after it has been in place for a while, she feels increasingly listless and her sexual desire vanishes. So out comes the IUD. Her cheerfulness and interest in sex return.

In both instances, when contraception was stopped, the troublesome symptoms rapidly disappeared. But hormones cannot be blamed for the discomfort Mrs. Jones experienced. The answer to many women's difficulties with birth control lies partly in their less obvious feelings about the methods used, feelings which they often keep secret or try to push out of awareness. But, more significantly, these emotions extend beyond contraception to all aspects of childbearing. For instance, if a woman believes that being a mother is enjoyable and important, and a basic part of her sexuality, then a contraceptive which denies her the chance to become pregnant may affect her well-being and self-esteem. Though she may *think* she wants a contraceptive, it actually makes her feel sexless and useless. Some women tend then to feel guilty about having sexual intercourse "for no purpose." When such a woman takes the pill, she thinks she's doing something wrong and expects that she will be punished. She may think she will become ill, or that she will become pregnant anyway and miscarry. In fact, if there are clots in the menstrual blood, she may misinterpret this to mean that a miscarriage is actually occurring. She clings to these ideas, even though she has been emphatically told in advance that the pill will have no such effect.

Neither Mrs. Smith nor Mrs. Jones really wanted birth control. Mrs. Smith already had two children but she also had a powerful, though hidden, need to become a mother repeatedly. She was the youngest and only girl among four children. Her brothers banded together, excluding her. Her father was always doing things with the boys, without her. Her mother, pretty, vivacious, and the one who ran things in that family, was the center of male attention. So, as a little girl, Mrs. Smith felt quite neglected. She surrounded herself with dolls, and her favorite game was playing house. Later she daydreamed that when she grew up she would be like her mother, adored by a husband and many children. Her envy of her mother, though it faded out of awareness as she grew up, never actually left her. In her teens, all she could think about was getting married. Her early marriage to a successful lawyer was for her a special triumph. Thus far she felt she had done better than her mother. But she wasn't satisfied; deep inside she also felt she needed a big family. Then, after two children, she paused, wondering if she had the energy, the emotional reserves, to add more. So she turned to the pill. But even as she took it, her inner emotions told her she really didn't want to put a stop to childbearing. She was not given the chance at the clinic to reveal any of this, which would have signaled that she was poorly motivated for birth control.

Rationally Mrs. Jones didn't want any more children. She already had five, and things were rough in the marriage. Her husband, a taxi driver and would-be writer, rarely spent time with her and the children. When not out at his job, he would bury himself in an attic room among a clutter of rejected manuscripts. Every once in a while he had sex with her, but it was quick and mechanical; he was done long before she felt able to achieve a climax. The care and upbringing of the children was left entirely to her. More additions to the family seemed to be out of the question. So she was fitted for an IUD. But in addition to being a neglected, frustrated wife, she didn't make friends easily. For her, being surrounded by many children, even in a rotten marriage, was a compensation which prevented her from becoming lonely or depressed. She, too, had no opportunity to unburden herself of these indicators at the clinic.

Thus, though seemingly wanting birth control, both women deep down could not tolerate the idea that they would not become pregnant. And this is frequently an important, contributory reason why many other women also suffer peculiar reactions to contraceptives. Often, too, the attitude of the husband can initiate or reinforce the wife's unconscious rejection of contraceptives.

What other psychological signs are there that indicate contraceptives are apt to fail or produce unpleasant symptoms? One is a strong desire for children in young women, even though they outwardly say they want more years of "freedom." Another is that some couples think sterility, even though it is artificially produced, is degrading. A man may suffer from this feeling, and thus make his wife feel tense, or the feeling may originate with the wife herself. Women, or couples, who feel it's sinful to have sexual relations just for pleasure will be uneasy with contraception. Still other women will reject contraception if their marriage is marred by sexual incompatibility; they seek to avoid intercourse, and birth control deprives them of the excuse that sex might get them pregnant. They fear their husbands can ask, even demand, sex any time with contraception. Women forced by their husbands to practice birth control will tolerate it poorly.

Some wives are so immobilized and so apathetic because of the terrible poverty their families are mired in that they simply can't adhere to any plan. So even though they have many children, can't afford to have any more, and seek contraceptive advice, they can't follow it. Certain women, very concerned about their physical well-being, are afraid the use of an IUD or the pill will have serious effects on their bodies and may even cause that most dreaded of consequences—cancer. All of these women stop contraception or become careless about it. So when a couple has difficulty with birth control, the course of their problem can very often be found in the attitudes of the husband, or wife, or both, rather than in the contraceptive itself.

What indicates good motivation for birth control? Real enjoyment of sexual relations and full agreement between wife and husband that the first or next child should be postponed. Women who have had children, and who feel fulfilled in their roles as wife and mother, also will have no trouble with birth control. Their husbands are not likely to. be concerned about potency, so their attitudes will be positive also, and they will not make their wives feel guilty or sexless over it. Surprisingly, though, healthy, positive attitudes toward sex and motherhood are not the only prerequisites for successful contraception. Sometimes *negative* attitudes toward sex and motherhood indicate such an outcome. A woman who is afraid of pregnancy and childbirth, and who has visions she will suffer terrible complications, may look on contraception as a lifesaver, and so she has no trouble with it. Others who adapt well to birth control wish to avoid having their figures misshaped. For them the baby inside is like a parasite. And such attitudes may be reinforced by a husband who, perhaps because he has to prop up his self-confidence by showing off a ravishing wife, also wishes his wife's body to remain unchanged. Or the husband may want his wife all to himself and be unable to share her with a child. Then there are women, or couples, who feel even one or two children are too much for them, and they welcome birth control eagerly.

I think that you will have gathered from some of the above that the husband's attitude toward birth control cannot be disregarded. When the attitude is positive, or at least neutral—and in agreement with the wife's reaction—birth control will be most successful. The man often feels relieved of the responsibility for his wife's becoming pregnant when she uses contraceptives. However, it may come as a great surprise to him if he assumes she's practicing birth control and then suddenly she announces one day that she is pregnant. This happened to one of my patients. He had been married several years but he and his wife were having problems. They had agreed not to have children, since a divorce seemed inevitable. After this understanding, the husband turned to several other women. Relations between husband and wife became even more strained and sexual intercourse rarer. She bitterly resented his attentions to other women and insisted the marriage had to be terminated. However, they were both unaware that a neurotic pattern had been stirred up in her, making her feel she would be unwanted by anyone if her husband abandoned her. So neither of them understood why she suddenly became "careless" about contraception. It was simply that without being aware of it she hoped a pregnancy would save the marriage. So there they were, ready for divorce and faced with the question of what to do about an unexpected baby.

Some men who interpret their wives' pregnancies and number of babies as evidence of their own virility will become emotionally disturbed if the wife insists on birth control. Other men, locked into an incompatible marriage because of neurotic reasons, vent their hostility in an unusual way: the more their wives protest against additional children, the more the husbands insist that they become pregnant. Should the wife try to practice contraception, the husband, frustrated in his attempt to impregnate her, may accuse her of wanting to be unfaithful and may even beat her up for thwarting him.

Though conflict contributes to the difficulties you may experience when you practice birth control, doctors still tend to dispense contraceptive advice without evaluating your emotional state and the clues it gives to future trouble. And that trouble may be in the form of severe physical complications. One such is the highly publicized thromboembolic condition (blood clots) associated with the estrogen hormone in the conventional pill. Other complications include migraine, stomach upsets, and high blood pressure. But these undesirable side effects do not occur in every woman taking the pill, nor are they exclusively due to its chemical effect. A woman's bodily functions also may be disrupted by severe emotional strain. The disturbance then can be local—the reproductive organs being the target area—or it can be systemic (general). The pill changes hormonal balance, suppressing the ovulatory phase of the woman's cycle. But the estrogen in the pill also seems to play a role in the formation of blood clots. This effect could be enhanced by emotion which can cause all kinds of hormonal and vascular disturbances. If you're under great tension, it behooves you to think of your feelings and consult with a physician who takes them into consideration. If they reveal signs of vulnerability to bodily disorder, you'll be less apt to tell yourself that contraceptive pills are as easy as swallowing aspirin.

That's not what Corinne did. She was a seemingly happy-go-lucky woman in her early forties whose two children had both just left home to further their careers. Her husband missed them and openly showed his depression. But she seemed to take their leaving in stride. It was at this time that Corinne decided that the diaphragm she had been using was an awkward contraceptive device. The doctor whom the family occasionally had consulted about health problems put her on the pill when she told him over the phone she wanted to change. Some weeks later Corinne, who had a part-time job as a saleswoman, began to notice that her right leg felt stiff and painful while she was at work. This continued, but Corinne, as was her habit when she experienced any discomfort, paid no attention to her leg, didn't even look at it. One evening, just as she got home and stood on the threshold thinking how empty it all seemed, an agonizing pain exploded in her chest. She could hardly breathe, her legs buckled, and she fell to the floor. At the hospital the doctors told her she had a blood clot in her right lung. The clot had been thrown off from an inflammation of veins (thrombophlebitis) in her right leg.

Corinne was quite ill and for the first time in her memory felt worried about herself. A consultant discovered that she habitually denied anything unpleasant and had been trying to deny her feeling of emptiness and grief ever since her children, to whom she was very attached, had left. How to fill the void? She tried more sexual activity with her husband, but it wasn't really satisfying—it never had been. Attempts to avoid her feelings by working harder were ineffective. Bitterness at their leaving her was pushed almost immediately out of mind. Troublesome dreams of being alone and unable to care for herself were quickly repressed, as were recollections of being separated from her mother who had been hospitalized for tuberculosis. What were all these? Psychological signs that her body was being wracked by a great strain and that it had been the wrong time to start on the pill.

Similarly, though the insertion of an IUD is a minor procedure, after it's in place, physical and psychological complications can occur. Personal fears about the consequences of using an IUD may be great, e.g., that it will cause cancer or ruin future fertili·y, and some women have the extraordinary fantasy that if pregnancy occurs despite the IUD and then goes on to term, the infant will be born with the device through its nose or ear.

But how can we tell whether physical complications will occur in women who plan to use an IUD? The following are signs: (1) a sensitized uterus because of past experiences, so that it is a target organ which malfunctions when the woman is subject to great stress; (2) a history of recent emotional trauma with few psychological outlets for the accumulated tension; (3) conflicts about becoming pregnant; (4) recurrent fantasies of being violated or mutilated; (5) frequent thoughts about relatives or friends who have had gynecological·difficulties.

Irrespective of what contraceptive device is being considered, in every instance the *emotional* as well as the physical state of both wife and husband bear careful scrutiny. Psychological clues elicited at such times are valuable aids in forecasting possible trouble with contraception. Counseling or more formal therapy may then be indicated.

WHEN TO EXPECT STERILIZATION COMPLICATIONS

Vasectomy, which sterilizes men, or tubal ligation, which sterilizes women, are both simple surgical procedures. However, neither should be done on impulse or whim, without careful consideration of your current emotional state. Though sterilization may lessen tensions, this is not necessarily so; in fact, the opposite may occur. It is not a magical solution for marital problems. One unfortunate sequel can be depression—foreshadowed prior to operation by (1) the patient's tenacious belief that the ability to impregnate or conceive is the sign of adequacy as a person, and (2) the patient's preoccupation with losing masculine or feminine appeal. Other consequences predictable from these clues, together with evidence of activated self-destructive impulses and blocking of psychological outlets, are postoperative physical complications: infection or slow healing of the wound; "mysterious" disorders of the genito-urinary tract—sometimes immediately or after a delay of weeks or months; and other body disorders.

SEX AND CHRONIC ILLNESS

There is still another aspect of sexual influence on the body to be considered. Suppose you have already had a physical illness and have been left with a chronic disability. Can you tell whether sexual activity will have an adverse effect on your condition?

If you have heart trouble or high blood pressure and are considering extramarital sex, it would be wise to take note of the following. Are you experiencing unusual anticipatory anxiety about *how* you will perform and unusual anticipatory guilt over *what* you will be doing? Or do you have no feelings at all about it? If the answer is yes either way, the chances are that overt or concealed emotional upset will worsen your physical condition. The risk factor is heightened if the sexual activity is preceded by a heavy meal and alcohol. On the other hand, if you're a long-married cardiac living compatibly with your spouse, and if you engage in marital sex, there will tend to be no physical complications. But, in an incompatible marriage, attempts at sexual contact with your spouse, accompanied by frustration, a buildup of intense hostility which is largely repressed, together with guilt which seems to disappear may also be followed by aggravation of your bodily ailment. When you have a chronic illness or are subject to recurrent bodily ailments and are getting a checkup, a survey of your emotional state should include your sexual desires and conflicts. This may clearly reveal important indicators of possible physical complications if you are contemplating sexual activity.

In each and every one of us, our emotions affect our sexual life and our sexual activities affect our emotions. Both affect the way our bodies work and are prime indicators of whether we will be healthy or sick. If we know something about these and heed the warnings they give us, we can prevent or lessen physical disorders associated with sexuality—disorders which, once they are well established, are generally difficult to treat.

15

Psychological Warnings of Infection

Are there psychological signs that forewarn us of infectious disease? This may seem an odd question to those who think of such illness in purely physical terms. They would argue that specific bacteria and viruses have been demonstrated for most infections, that laboratory tests can determine immunity, and that key factors in prevention and treatment are eradication of disease vectors and use of protective vaccines and chemicals. Infectious-disease specialists usually want a specific kind of information—they would ask what contact we have had with infected humans, animals, insects or food, milk, water, needles. But it is also true that germs on or even in our bodies will not necessarily make us sick.

TB OR NOT TB

Some years ago I saw a number of veterans who had contracted tuberculosis in POW camps and whose recovery was slow and complicated, with frequent relapses. TB, of course, as we have all been taught, is caused by a specific bacillus. Yet in talking with these men, I wondered why they had come down with the illness while other POWs who were exposed to the bacilli did not contract the disease. I also wondered why their response to treatment had been so poor. Now as I think back to those interviews with the tubercular POWs, I realize that from the details of the emotional upheaval these men had gone through, one also could have elicited the signs which foretold that they would get sick. They had reacted to imprisonment by becoming withdrawn and apathetic. They felt their loss of status keenly, and their morale was poor. All their anger had become bottled up and turned against themselves. A number of them had received news of relatives' becoming ill or dying. Others had fantasies and dreams of withering away. Finally, feelings of helplessness and hopelessness had descended on them, to be followed by TB. This only reinforced their gloomy mood and lessened their will to live.

So we see that limited capacity to adapt to severe emotional trauma, poor morale, pent-up hostility, activated self-destructive impulses, inadequate psychological outlets, identification with sick or dead relatives, and disturbing dreams are all indicators of susceptibility to infection and slowness of recovery.

These signs are valid in all kinds of situations, peacetime as well as wartime. Previously they were not known, or at least they were not used. Instead only the most general references to emotion were made, and then as causal factor rather than predictor. A high death rate from tuberculosis struck down Navajo and Sioux Indians who were being shifted from one reservation to another and also immigrants coming from the farms of Ireland to the cities of America at the turn of the century. In both instances it was noted only that these people were subjected to great psychological pressures as they tried to adapt to a new environment. Apart from tuberculosis, it is well known that epidemics of infectious disease in general tend to occur during periods of massive upheaval in the lives of people. What war can do to familiar surroundings and routines we all know. But environmental ravages also occur during times of so-called peace when racism, unemployment, oppression, and poverty affect millions. When things aren't going right over and over again for the community (or larger sections of the population), for the family, and for the individual, the emotional equilibrium of many people will be shaken. But it is only when the emotional makeup of each person is examined that the specific psychological indications of vulnerability to infectious disease become more evident; moreover, such a psychological examination can reveal where the vulnerability will manifest itself.

PRELUDE TO MUMPS

So epidemics do not affect everyone who is exposed to the rampaging germs. Even the infectious diseases of childhood run different courses in different individuals. Some children who contract measles and chicken pox have what is called subclinical infections and are hardly ill; others become very sick and develop dangerous complications. Still others do not contract the illness until they become adults.

Consider the following case. Mrs. Peters, a sophisticated thirty-five-year-old suburbanite, had never had mumps. Nevertheless, when her older son, a boy of six, came down with it, she nursed him herself. The child was headstrong and rebellious. He had often given her a hard time, and usually she had not been able to control her anger at him. Now she wanted to make up for her impatience with him. She knew he had guessed that she favored his younger brother (a compliant, model child), who also developed mumps but in a very mild form and was hardly sick. Strangely, Mrs. Peters did not come down with it, despite her sustained contact with the children. The hidden facts were that her gentler behavior toward the older boy was neutralizing her hostility and guilt.

A year went by, and she became involved in a legal struggle with her father over details of an estate left by her mother, who had died of cancer. Mrs. Peters did not feel her usual self at all. She had hardly mourned her mother's passing, but frequently thought of her mother's cancer. Toward her father she felt a strange apathy, despite their disagreements. One Sunday while the controversy over the will was still unsettled, she took her two boys to a birthday party, staying only for a brief chat with the hostess. Several children at the party developed mumps later, and she was relieved that her boys had already had this illness. But she herself continued to feel under par. Her neck seemed to her to be drawn and stiff. She had a number of dreams about little animals. One in particular left a vivid impression. It pictured baby kangaroos jumping in and out of their mother's pouch. Mrs. Peters' own dependency needs were being strongly activated as her psychological equilibrium shifted (regressively) under the impact of emotional pressures that seemed to be going under cover. Was the development of a body disturbance also being signaled?

Some weeks later her husband remarked that the right side of her face appeared swollen. Not mumps, was her first thought. That would be more than ironic, indeed incomprehensible, when she had had practically no contact with anyone at the party. After all, a year previously, though she had been exposed to the illness in her own children, nothing had happened to her. There was a difference, however, but she was unaware of its significance. *Then,* her emotional equilibrium had remained relatively stable. She felt *good.* She was being a devoted mother, nursing the children, and indeed the older boy, after recovering from his sickness, seemed to get along better with her. *Now* her body was being severely shaken by her hidden grief over her mother's death and her unresolved controversy with her father—feelings that had been blocked off from outward expression. And this time she indeed came down with mumps, even though the exposure was minimal.

MORE THAN MEETS THE EYE

The development of infectious illness, its complications, aftereffects, and the length of convalescence from it can be better estimated by studying psychological clues as well as the physical ones. It has been known for some time that mumps, measles, and other childhood infections tend to occur more often, and more severely, in a youngster exposed to constant family turmoil than in one living in a more tranquil setting. Similarly, infections are more apt to develop in the emotionally unstable adult. But these are generalizations. For purposes of prediction, it is far more useful to have as much detailed information as possible about specific psychological indicators of susceptibility to infection in each person. They signal that our immunological and antibody responses which fight off infection simply aren't going to work effectively. And they predict that changes in the body's chemical balance and in the blood supply of the tissues will occur which enable bacteria or viruses to take hold. In this case our nasal membranes will be so affected that breathing in a small amount of pollen (which causes no symptoms when we're not under tension) may produce a severe attack of hay fever. Recent research indicates that lowered resistance not only to infection, but also to rheumatoid arthritis and even to cancer, is related to disturbed immunological responses of the body—which in turn may be forecast by a continuing emotional imbalance.

Let us turn to another case. Faith, a twenty-four-year-old nursery school teacher, engaged to be married, went about her work wrapped in a romantic haze, her mind busy with wedding plans. Then her fiancé was called out of town on a business trip. Though he had phoned her regularly, she began to feel uneasy when he told her one evening that he would be away longer than expected because his company was sending him immediately to South America. But he promised that he would write all the details.

It was an unusually humid spring afternoon when the postman brought the letter. It was quiet in the playroom. Earlier, even the nursery children had seemed subdued, and some were absent because they had come down with German measles which had been going around the community for a month. She stared unbelievingly at the scrawl in front of her. There was another girl, and they had flown to Rio together. The engagement was off, and he hoped Faith would understand. Bold, blunt, brutal. Her bitter anger was replaced by feelings of humiliation and helplessness. Friends tried to console her without success. She sought to escape in a flurry of projects for her pupils.

But intrusive thoughts about the loss of her fiancé kept plaguing her. And there was more. She had skipped a period and began to wonder if she were pregnant. Her friends said *that* was due to psychological shock, so Faith tried to dismiss all emotion from her mind. For some weeks she was so busy with schoolwork that she had no time to think about her problems or feel anything at all—consciously, that is. Under the surface, it was different: emotions were seething in her; rage and despair were threatening to blow the lid off. They finally did. One night a bad dream about being run down by a fire engine woke her screaming with fright. Then, for a fleeting moment she had the thought: "Something terrible is going to happen to my body." This was the final clue in a series that had been warning of impending physical trouble. The next day she went to her gynecologist, and the first thing he noticed was a faint red rash all over her body. She was coming down with German measles. And after further examination he made a second diagnosis—yes, she was pregnant. And under the worst possible circumstances. The new life within her was threatened with deformity by the virus she was harboring. Fortunately, a safe and legal abortion saved Faith from further tragedy. But the fact remains that she, like Mrs. Peters, though exposed to disease, had not contracted it until her upset emotions affected her resistance. And neither woman had understood the significance of the signals which presaged this outcome.

COURTING INFECTION

At other times, it seems that we are being impelled to court an infection. For instance, take the case of Alfred, a handsome but shy college sophomore, and Marilyn, the seductive senior he met at a mixer. Troubled by inferiority feelings, Alfred had spent his first year at school grinding away at his studies, living like a recluse. He was frightened silly when he thought of competing with the big jocks, or the big brains. He persuaded himself that no girl would prefer him to them. Sex for him was masturbation, in which he pictured himself an irresistible man-about-campus. The strain of loneliness finally forced him to go to this mixer—his very first—but along with him went his constant companion, anxiety. And what about Marilyn? Even though she told him she had a nagging sore throat, that staying in bed hadn't done any good, and that she'd figured a party might be just the medicine she needed, Alfred wasn't about to turn down such a fascinating girl just because she had some germ. He was so nervous that he might not kiss her properly that even later, when they were in her apartment, he was a lot more worried about how he was performing than he was about what might be wrong with her. He even joked that it might be "mono" which his sister had had the previous year—the sore throat, painful glands in the neck, the dragging fatigue that seemed to go on forever. A tiny alarm bell did go off in his mind when Marilyn said that she felt just like his sister had. But it wasn't enough to lessen his pent-up

longing and make him pass over the chance to prove he
was the man-about-campus he'd dreamed of being. Those
needs, greatly activated, were the signs that he was on the
verge of becoming reckless and disregarding reality. And
that's what happened. The night was given over to passionate
kissing, petting, and naked contact.

The following afternoon Alfred got a call from Marilyn.
She was in the infirmary with infectious mononucleosis. He
rushed over to see her, and every day he spent as much
time as he could with her, until he came down with the
same thing.

So when we are blue, when inferiority feelings bug us,
and when there is the chance for a relationship—sexual or
otherwise—with someone who is desirable but may have
an infectious disease, then our judgment may not be clear
and objective. Those are warnings that we are susceptible
to infection, not only because stress has lowered our resistance, but also because our feelings have made us toss caution
aside. Though we may blame a germ, emotion has hit us
two ways.

This is not the only circumstance in which we can suffer
physically because of our hangups. If we are troubled by
a bad conscience, we may unconsciously try to atone by
punishing ourselves—by doing something that will hurt us.
Suppose I'm under stress, lose my temper, and rage at my
family. Afterward I feel a little guilty, but I'm not quite
ready to give in and apologize. All this is a sign of trouble
to come. Then I cut my finger "accidentally" as I carve
the roast for dinner. Ordinarily I would take care of such
a cut, putting an antiseptic and bandage on it. But this time
I rationalize: I'm not going to give up the façade of a tough
guy in a cool, controlled rage by suddenly turning into a
cry baby who needs his finger bandaged. I neglect the cut.
And it blossoms into a nasty infection. So I not only hurt
myself because of a bad conscience, I let my emotional state
complicate my injury.

In many similar situations, when your emotions are upset, you will find yourself taking chances and disregarding warnings to be careful. These are indications that you may expose yourself to situations that are potentially dangerous to your health as well as your reputation. Sexual frustration is an example of the sort of emotional pressure that may interfere with good judgment. Say you're married but no longer enjoy sex with your spouse, or single and dissatisfied with all the women (men) you know—and you decide an orgy is just what you need to shake you out of your rut. You're not likely to be deterred by worry over careless sexual contact. In fact, you've probably drowned any qualms in alcohol or drugs, so any worries you had seem plain silly. Strep throats, infectious mononucleosis, cold sores (which can cause severe mouth and throat infections), other infections, and of course, venereal diseases—all can be transmitted under these circumstances.

Interestingly, it's not just the victim who has an emotional hangup. Often the person who transmits the infection—say, a venereal disease—does not pass it on through ignorance, but because of hostility. Sometimes that person is not aware of his or her hidden motives for doing so, is not aware that exposing someone else to infection is a way of expressing anger. At other times such people are quite conscious of what they are doing. They may even think it is some kind of justifiable revenge: "She said she was clean and I trusted her. So I got the syph. She's just like all the others—a dirty, deceiving whore. I'm getting treatment, but I'm not going to tell that to any broad who wants a piece. Let her take her chances." This sort of deliberate desire to hurt someone else comes from a very disturbed person. For this reason, in a random sexual encounter, you should not only be aware of the physical risks involved, but you should also consider whether your partner is emotionally upset.

Salmonella is the cause of a very common gastrointestinal infection in humans. At least two million people in this country alone become ill from it annually, particularly during the warm months when the germ multiplies rapidly. It is found in pet turtles, as well as in various meats, poultry, and especially cracked eggs, which if insufficiently cooked may cause symptoms of what is called food poisoning: nausea, vomiting, bellyache, and diarrhea. While most adults weather the sickness without difficulty except for brief, acute distress, the outcome may be more serious for babies, chronically ill individuals, and those whose gut has become a target organ, who are ready to explode with anger but can't, and so have a greater than usual need to suffer.

Psychological forces also tend to make us more susceptible to the deadly germs of cholera and typhoid. If we are headed for an area where the disease is endemic, and are aware that some of these psychological susceptibilities are present in us, we need to take special care to protect ourselves—by inoculations, careful personal hygiene, and above all, some reduction of our tension.

FOOLING THE PIGS

A recent study of the salmonella germ was done on a pig farm. Tests for salmonella (done by examining stools) were negative as long as the pigs lived quietly in their habitual surroundings. However, after they were driven to the slaughterhouse, many were found to have the disease. Previously, it had remained hidden and inactive in their intestines until they were subjected to transport, overcrowding, and rough handling. Then bowel and bacterial activity increased. In another part of the experiment, pigs were taken for a ride through the pleasant countryside, but this time the trip ended back at the farm. Had the pigs been fooled? They had reacted to the "joy ride" as if they were going to the slaughterhouse. In each instance transport and overcrowding were stressful, and bacteria were found in the stools.

Other experiments have shown that purging will result

in the flushing of cholera organisms from their hiding place in the upper gut or gallbladder, and in their appearance in the stools. As we have seen, stress may have the same effect as purging. So cholera carriers are more apt to spread the disease when psychological signs indicate such persons are under severe tensions.

WHEN WILL YOU GET A COLD?

An outbreak of cholera or typhoid or plague makes dramatic headlines. But a less exotic illness—the common cold—affects tens of millions of people every year. It can cause total misery, disruption of plans, and staggering economic loss. Germs, as well as immunological response, antibody formation, and other protective mechanisms of the body, have been the focus of research into this affliction. Air pollutants have been implicated. Although people realize that nervousness is related to colds, they are not always aware of the specific psychological clues that often precede upper respiratory infections.

Everybody has had a bad cold at one time or another. Yet how many of us recall the precise emotional state that preceded our last cold? Perhaps all we can remember is that there was an epidemic of flu that missed very few people. One year we escape, another year we join the many victims. If we came down with it, is it possible that we had more exposure than people who escaped? Were we perhaps less immune? Or is it more likely that our emotions contributed to needless exposure, to lessened immunity, or to the need to just get away from the rat race and rest in bed for a few days? What was going on before you noticed a runny nose? Were you studying for an exam, about to take an unwelcome trip, or returning from one? Were you reluctantly preparing for a public appearance, facing a social engagement you didn't relish? Had you just quarreled, had a hard time at work or with your family? Were you about to move to another residence or take a new job? A new baby coming? These are all stress situations.

There are other indicators. Had something happened with which you couldn't cope, or about which you had to hold back your real feelings? Had there been a buildup of hostility? Was there evidence that something might have depressed you? Were you trying—successfully—to shut all unplesantness out of your conscious thinking? Were colds a habitual way you responded to unusual psychological pressures? Do you have a severe conscience, ready to make you suffer one way or another? Is someone else among your relatives and friends subject to many colds, and do you strongly identify with that person?

Good examples of emotional pressures that reduce resistance to upper respiratory infections—colds, tonsillitis, pharyngitis, laryngitis, bronchitis, and sinusitis—can be found among college students and young people entering military service. Both groups come from all parts of the country and face a new way of life. Old adaptive patterns may be severely tested, and perhaps can't be used. New ways are substituted, sometimes in the form of acting out (violent behavior, drugs, AWOL), more often in a somatization response—getting sick physically. These responses represent regressive shifts in psychological equilibrium. Difficulties in ventilating feelings, particularly rage—especially against Establishment figures—are common to both groups. Dependency needs are often frustrated just when they are most stirred up by the new environment. Those with self-punitive tendencies will be even more subject to upper respiratory infections and other illnesses.

The student and the soldier who go to the infirmary are often signaling that they're desperate for a chance to talk about their "other troubles," even though they might not be aware that this was really the reason. If the doctor is understanding and kind, he'll try to help them let off some steam. He might be able to give them some guidance or direct them to it. But many students and soldiers keep their troubles to themselves. And, not heeding the psychological as well as physical signs that their health is in jeopardy, they may try to sidestep their troubles until a dangerous illness may result.

Infections are indeed caused by specific germs. But whether we become susceptible to them depends to a certain extent on our psychological state.

16

Emotions That Foretell Tooth Trouble

Are our teeth affected by our emotions? Up until about twenty-five years ago practically everybody, including dentists, would have been amazed that such a question was even being asked. After all, a tooth is a bonelike structure, hard, used for biting and chewing, which can be scraped at and drilled into, or even extracted.

But teeth have a nerve supply and a blood supply. They are bathed constantly by saliva and periodically in contact with all kinds of food and drink—sometimes with fingers, cigarettes, cigars, pipes, pencils, or pens—and less often with other mouths and other parts of other bodies. We sometimes show our anger by baring our teeth and grinding them; biting is the original form of this emotional response in little children. A voluptuous, sexually attractive woman is described as toothsome. When we talk of a special taste or appetite for certain foods, we refer to a sweet tooth. The expression "armed to the teeth" signifies complete preparation for attack. When we want to indicate that we are actively involved, that we have a firm grasp of something, we say we've gotten our teeth into it. Our mouths and teeth are indeed related, not only physically but psychologically, to the rest of us. Our mouths are, in fact, one of the most erotic areas of the entire body as well as a vehicle for expressing angry feelings. Directly or indirectly, and symbolically, they reflect all our passions. And similarly, our passions are reflected in the condition of our mouths and our teeth.

SPECIFIC SIGNS

There are psychological clues to impending disorder in this part of our body, but we have to be on the lookout for them, because they're elusive. Some people express anger by clenching their jaws and grinding their teeth, both during the day and during sleep at night. Some of us show our tension by chewing on almost anything we can get hold of. The more needy we feel, the more we may use our mouths, lick our lips, suck, and salivate.

Signs of developing dental trouble can also be found in our waking fantasies and in our dreams. Ideas of biting people, even cannibalistic thoughts—common in children and later ordinarily repressed—may flash through consciousness when we as adults feel especially deprived and frustrated. But we have to be on the alert to detect them among the many other fantasies crowding our minds. It will be especially hard to pick these "oral" fantasies out if you're a "doer" and not a "thinker."

Excessive, unusual preoccupation with food and eating may sometimes signal the onset of teeth and mouth problems. Behind this preoccupation is an excessive urge to bite, which is then camouflaged by actual overactivity in chewing when we eat. When fellatio and cunnilingus stir up sadistic impulses, is there anxiety and guilt? If these are briefly conscious and then disappear, this may indicate the development of mouth disorders.

Our dreams, activated by "oral" conflicts, may, at times, presage dental trouble in a clearly symbolic fashion. Here's an example. Two rows of soldiers stand facing one another, then attack each other, then resume their original position.

This goes on until one falls wounded or dead. We may wake up with a toothache, or develop one in a few days.

Still another sign is a hostile relationship with someone who has had or is having dental problems. Self-destructive tendencies result in lack of care of the body—in this instance, the mouth and its structures. Under these circumstances, if dental disease is already present, nothing will be done about it. Persuasive or pressuring tactics by relatives or friends will be resisted. Denial, if prominent in the thinking and utterances of the person with mouth disorder, is another indication that proper treatment will be avoided, because "there's nothing wrong."

Certain habits such as grinding the teeth (bruxism)—often accompanied by jaw movements of which we may be unaware—cheek biting, excessive chewing of food and gum, or biting or chewing on fingernails, pencils, pens, or pipes, all have psychological meanings. Often we do these things out of a craving for oral (mouth) satisfactions, and from anger when this need is frustrated. At the same time, incessant biting and chewing put a strain on the tissues and structures surrounding and supporting our teeth. If we continue to be upset and keep grinding our teeth or sucking and chewing on things, we can cause constriction of the blood vessels supplying the gums and bone in which teeth are set. As a result, there will be an inadequate supply of oxygen and other essential nutrients, and diseases can develop in the gums, bones, and teeth.

And just as being upset can lower our resistance to infection in other parts of our body, this also applies to various infections of the mouth. If you have a lot of anxiety that cannot find adequate release in your feelings and behavior, then it may hit your body in predisposed areas, including your mouth. A study done on students preparing for exams showed that in those who were very nervous *and* had poor mouth hygiene, a condition known as Vincent's angina (trench mouth) occurred. Tension and neglect of teeth also lead to trench mouth in military recruits or in men facing combat for the first time. Finally, we know that very tense people suffer more infection of the bony structures around the teeth than do relaxed people. In any event, the mouth is part of our body and influenced by the same emotions as the rest of it. Although dentistry has been a separate health science, in recent years dental education and medical education have tended to merge more and more. But recognition of the role that our feelings play in dental conditions lags far behind.

DENTISTRY BLOCKED

Some people ignore dental hygiene and treatment, don't brush their teeth, and fail to visit the dentist until severe pain or infection forces them to seek treatment. This type of procrastination often has childhood origins. All of us, as children, suffered some degree of pain when our teeth began to erupt from the gums. Depending on other factors, particularly how your parents handled you during this trying time, you may be conditioned to disregard the condition of your mouth or teeth later on. If your parents were not comforting or, in fact, tended to pay little attention to you, you might have interpreted the discomfort of losing your baby teeth as a kind of punishment; as a result, later you might not want to admit that anything is wrong with your teeth that would require their treatment or removal (because that would symbolically mean you had done something for which you were to be punished).

Your first experience with dentists is also going to play a part in your adult attitudes. If your childhood dentist was unpleasant or made you afraid, you might as an adult continue to fear being terribly hurt. You will then see dental procedures as dreadful, to be avoided at almost any cost. Under these circumstances your dentist may even come to represent an ogre, awakening old fears of punishment for things you said or did, things you knew adults would not approve of (usually sexual or hostile). If you are inclined to be a highly self-punitive, guilt-ridden person, you will, without being aware of it, behave in ways that hurt you needlessly, and among other disservices to yourself you will neglect your teeth even when they obviously require attention and treatment.

CHILDHOOD EXPERIENCES WITH DENTISTS

How sensitive or insensitive our parents and dentists were to us as children therefore has long-range implications. Some youngsters are accustomed to having few or no limits set to their behavior. Their mothers are apt to be passive, anxious, and simply unable to control their child's chaotic, dominating, disruptive behavior in the dentist's office. In these instances a firm approach by the dentist may be just what is needed. However, many children, who are quite naturally nervous about the new experience of having dental work done, may come up against a strong-arm dentist. Even if his technical skill enables him to do the right thing dentally, his strong-arm approach may affect the fearful child for years to come. A dentist who smiles and then hurts a child without warning is not easily forgotten. Can you recall from childhood that time when the grinning, white-coated stranger with one hand held behind his back approached you in that dental chair, and at the last moment flashed the hidden forceps in front of your horrified eyes? Did you as a child have a dentist who put his hand or a towel over your mouth or even shut off your breathing for a moment to "control" your emotional upset? Such a dentist may get a tooth extracted or a filling done, but at a long-term cost. Children who have had these forced, unpleasant experiences may, as adults who can no longer be coerced, shy away from anything to do with dental hygiene or treatment. I have seen a number of such patients whose teeth and gums were in dreadful shape because they were too scared to have anyone work on their mouths.

The dentist who understands the frightened child, who is sympathetic and kind, can afford to wait and not use force. So if the procedure isn't done today, it'll be done tomorrow or next week. If it isn't a real emergency (and it rarely is), there's no realistic need to hurry. Gentleness and tactful, firm persuasiveness—even if it means a delay in treatment—will achieve a most important long-term goal: it will encourage the child's trust in dentists and dental care, a trust that will stand him in good stead later on.

During World War II a particular cartoon had an extraordinary circulation in the armed forces both in this country and abroad. It shows a male patient in a dental chair, with the dentist standing beside him. Firmly gripped in a forceps held by the dentist is a molar that apparently has just been extracted. Connected to the tooth by cords and dangling from it is a complete set of male sex organs. Both patient and dentist are looking at this in horrified amazement. This cartoon, circulated mostly among men and generally enjoyed in a wry fashion, represents in a clear-cut way what the loss of a tooth means symbolically for many men. But the degree of emotional upset caused by extraction will vary considerably from man to man. To some men it is so sexually symbolic and frightening that they delay or refuse dental treatment. Other men seem hardly to care. Women also show a wide range of emotional reactions to loss of a tooth, some also not caring, while others feel they are being deprived of a vital part or being sexually assaulted.

Avoidance of the dentist is not necessarily due to emotional factors alone. Lack of money, insufficent dental health education, and the absence of low-cost clinics are other obstacles. But even if we get free dental care, it still might not be used by those of us who have been conditioned to fear pain, to see the dentist as policeman, judge, and high executioner.

Up until recent years, dentistry had been considered a profession in which technical skill and manual dexterity were the prime considerations. And many people felt that dental problems were a province outside the influence of emotion. But we have seen proof that emotional signs can predict dental disorders or the failure to have them treated. We also know that early conditioning has led us to become afraid of dentists or develop self-hurting tendencies. Prevention of such negative attitudes in childhood will do much to lessen the development of emotional blocks about dental hygiene and care when we become adults.

PART FOUR

Forecasting the Outcome of Illness

17

Psychological Reactions
to Bodily Change

How do we react when we *first* become aware of a bodily disorder? In different ways. Anxiously—expecting the worst; angrily—blaming others and holding them responsible for our illness; guiltily—as if we deserved what was happening to us. These are common responses. Many of us may try to avoid thinking of the physical symptoms or the emotions they evoke. Some feel hopeless and helpless. Few meet their physical problems calmly. *How* we respond emotionally can be as important as why our hangups triggered the illness to begin with. Each reaction is an indication of the course the disease may take and whether there will be interference either with our getting proper medical attention or with our recovery, or both.

AVOIDING TREATMENT

Suppose that you have a persistent headache but keep the concern to yourself until it becomes too much for you; then you have to share it with somebody else. You may do this directly, by informing friends that you can't get rid of this nagging pain. Or you may do it indirectly by pretending that a friend of yours has the headache, and wonder what it means or what can be done for your poor friend. So you tell the story in this disguised way to relatives, friends, neighbors, anyone who will listen, hoping they will offer suggestions. You'd probably pick on the local pharmacist, too, because he may sometimes suggest a patent medicine. Or you may be persuaded to buy the remedy guaranteed by radio or TV ads to bring relief. You may watch a TV medical show to see if any of the patients portrayed in it have your symptoms, what the diagnosis and treatment are, and whether the outcome is favorable. Or you may console yourself by thinking that all your ailments are due to "nerves." You'll do *anything* but go to your physician, because you're afraid the diagnosis will be horrible or that he will scold you, asking why you waited so long to get a checkup. Only when you get no relief and can stand the pain no longer will you finally seek medical help. If the headache turns out to be due to nervous tension, you could have spared yourself a lot of unnecessary suffering by consulting your physician earlier. But there's always the possibility that whatever is causing the headache is more serious and the delay has allowed it to progress to a truly dangerous point.

DENIAL

If denial is your response to bodily change, the problem is that you don't know you're denying anything. However, relatives, friends, health professionals may be able to spot this and help you become more aware of reality. Otherwise you can get into serious trouble. Consider the following instance where denial almost did the patient in. A man living alone has a hacking cough. He attributes this to his chain-smoking of cigarettes. But he doesn't seek medical advice because he can't give up the habit. And he can't give up the habit because it seems to make his troublesome tension a bit more tolerable. So he continues to smoke and continues to cough. In time a new symptom appears; he notices some shortness of breath. However, he doesn't bother to see his doctor about this either because, he explains to himself, *it* is the result of his sedentary life and lack of exercise. Actually he's trying to avoid the fear that an examination would reveal an incurable condition. His father recently died of tuberculosis. But after a few desultory attempts to be more active, he gives up all exercise, mostly because it makes his shortness of breath worse. As time goes by it becomes a struggle for him to breathe easily, even at rest. After several sleepless nights, sitting up in bed and gasping for air, he finally drags himself to a doctor. He has advanced emphysema, and it has progressed to a serious point. Thanks to hospitalization, an oxygen tent, and careful medical attention, he manages to stay alive. He had, of course, seen and heard about the effects of smoking, but his need to deny was working there too, just as it was in his refusal to seek early medical help.

SELF-DESTRUCTIVE BEHAVIOR AND ATONEMENT

Certain people, who are plagued by guilt and subject to self-destructive behavior, disregard these signs that their health will be threatened. Even when they become desperately ill, such people still do not ask for help. They finally may be brought to the hospital almost moribund, or else are found dead. I know of a student who kept secret the sudden appearance of blood in his stools. He had been ruminating about a car accident, in which he had injured an old man. He had such a severe conscience he couldn't stop blaming himself. Besides, deeply buried in his unconscious was a long-standing hatred of his own father, and guilt over *that*. Although the bloody stools persisted and, in addition, he developed bad stomach cramps, he didn't tell anybody. Even when the pain became excruciating, he bore it in silence, stuffing himself with aspirins. He became pale and haggard, suffering from constant pain and bloody diarrhea.

One night, sitting on the toilet, he keeled over in a dead faint. His roommate found him in a pool of blood, and in the hospital it was nip and tuck for a long time. That hemorrhage had drained him almost to the point of no return. He had ulcerative colitis, neglected, endured up to the last possible moment. Why? After he had injured the old man, he felt he was no good, even evil, and his illness seemed like a just punishment. To take care of himself, to get better, would have seemed almost like saying it was all right to hit the old man. So he suffered. It was a way of expressing how sorry he was, irrational though it might be—but that's how his conscience worked.

Children react strongly to illness, especially if they need to be hospitalized. However, many children do not get panicky and overactive, and thus the signs of psychological damage are not always obvious. Fear may practically paralyze many children emotionally, and they then become silent sufferers and are mistakenly considered to be undisturbed.

RELIGIOUS BELIEFS

Sometimes people use religious beliefs to avoid doctors or refuse medical or surgical procedures, even in life-and-death situations. A lonely, discouraged, middle-aged patient hurt her right leg in a fall. There was swelling and pain, but she didn't call a doctor, didn't get X-rayed. Her deeply religious beliefs persuaded her that healing and relief from oppressive feelings came from prayer, meditation, and faith. For a while she had trouble getting around, and neighbors helped out with the shopping and meals. Eventually the injury from the fall healed, but a large, tender spot remained just below the knee. After a month, a small lump appeared at this spot, and the pain got worse. Then the lump began to drain. Prayer, meditation, and faith had no effect on it. The leg felt weaker and weaker, and finally she could no longer stand on it. She had to stay in bed as feelings of weakness spread through her body. Even her religious advisers insisted that an exception had to be made and that she must consult a physician. The diagnosis was bone cancer, and amputation of her leg was imperative. She refused and died within a few months.

Few religions counsel their adherents to go this far in disregarding their bodies, but if people have private, compelling emotional needs requiring that they suffer and even die, their religious conviction may be used to excuse and conceal their self-destructive tendencies, signals of a bad outcome.

Lack of money is a frequent reason given for not seeking medical advice. This may be an alibi for avoiding such help because of neurotic anxiety, distrust, a need to suffer, or simple ignorance—even if clinical care is available at nominal fees or if hospitalization is paid through welfare. However, economic factors can't always be dismissed as a mere excuse, because inexpensive or free health facilities are in fact woefully inadequate in many communities, and poor people may choose the discomfort and even incapacity of illness rather than put up with cold or even hostile treatment at a "free" clinic. Often a deep feeling of humiliation drives the patient away from these sources of medical help, when he or she is subjected to a grueling means test or insensitive handling.

I have presented only a few of the many excuses we find for not going to our doctors when illness strikes, but they are among the most common and the ones we should watch for most, because they so often hide the emotional factors that are the real reason for deferring treatment. And these very psychological interferences are also signals that what otherwise might be a simple health problem will become complicated.

Incidentally, when a country has national health insurance, as many European countries do, people may take advantage of the opportunities for examination and treatment even when they are not physically ill. If they are upset or under a strain, bodily symptoms serve as a reason to go for medical consultation, when basically what such people really need is reassurance and emotional support. The time they get for this, however, is generally very brief. Nevertheless, whether health care is free or not, people, without being aware of it, often use a physical checkup as an opportunity to unburden themselves (if the doctor lets them), and it can be helpful, provided we do not rely on it exclusively, hoping it will cure deep and long-standing tensions.

So when we become ill, the first question to ask ourselves is, How are we reacting? Are we, like any of the people mentioned above, avoiding medical care?

THE RIGHT DOCTOR

Even if we recognize that we need a doctor, decide to do something about it, and pick one, how we get along with him or her is a most important indication—usually ignored—of what our adjustment to the illness will be like.

Today the trend is toward providing *more*, not necessarily *better*, medical care. Leading medical schools are concerned with delivering quality health care, with engineering techniques that will make such delivery more efficient. In fact, engineering schools and medical schools are collaborating for this purpose. That is fine if truly comprehensive medical services are provided. But when human beings who are sick are treated like machines that have broken down, and the emphasis is on more assembly lines and automation, a dangerous gap occurs in treatment because the sick person's feelings and the signs they afford about the course of the illness go unheeded. Instruments cannot understand our emotions or deal with them. This still has to be done by humans trained to recognize, and do something about, our emotional reactions to sickness, our recovery, and our subsequent state of health.

Where do we find such medical care? The old-time family doctor did not have the technical know-how of today's physician, but he knew his patients as people. He didn't have to explore their life situations or hangups. These he was well aware of because of his long-time, close relationship with his patients and their families, perhaps for three generations. Besides, his geographical location and his role in the community made him seem almost a member of many families—a warm, compassionate, perceptive member.

Ideally, nowadays we look for technically perfect, unfailingly considerate people to help us when we are sick. But the reality is that an approximation of this ideal is the best we can hope for. Not all doctors and other health professionals have the necessary technical competence, plus an understanding of the role that emotions play in illness and of the clues that they provide.

ANTICIPATING EMOTIONAL INTERFERENCE WITH TREATMENT

Once you acknowledge you have to see a doctor because of some symptom that is bothering you, and once you have found a good doctor, your troubles are not yet over. Because, surprisingly, it is not always easy to follow the doctor's advice—competent as it may be. Even though we may agree rationally that the course of treatment he prescribes is necessary, and even if we are able to swing it financially (or get financial assistance), our emotions may again interfere. Then, for all sorts of irrational reasons, we may decide to follow only part of the doctor's advice or not to follow it at all.

This is especially true when the regimen is to be in effect for any prolonged time, as in chronic illness.

You may be surprised to learn that when you are ill and upset, nongenital areas may assume sexual significance for you; then you'll see the insertion of instruments, needles, tubes, as sadistic—or perhaps seductive. There are medicines to be taken, diets, rules about exercise, rest, and checkups. Sticking to all these rules becomes a nuisance. What indicates how we will react to a treatment program? Some sick people whose habitual behavior is obsessional or who are passive follow recommendations to a "T." It may even become a ritual from which they get some gratification. Other patients keep a questioning check on all aspects of the treatment because they are so suspicious—even of their doctors. It is not unusual for such people to change doctors and treatments frequently. But many of us tend to be just a little careless or self-indulgent; we may not take a pill every three hours, or we may think *one* little helping of some forbidden food won't hurt, or engage in more strenuous activity than has been approved. This is common.

Others of us really sabotage the medical recommendations, consciously and unconsciously. We may not take the necessary medicine, because our need to punish ourselves and suffer is stronger than our desire to get well. In fact, if we are extremely self-destructive, we neglect medical advice altogether. At times, even if we have nothing against the doctor personally, stubborn contrariness may make us disregard some or all of his advice just because being ornery is part of our character.

A REBELLIOUS DIABETIC

When we find that we have some degree of resistance to medical advice—and most of us have *some*—we need a doctor who is aware of which psychological signals indicate a stormy course for the treatment. The right kind of doctor can make all the difference. Here's an example.

It was the third time in six months that Marty, only twenty years old, had been rushed to the emergency ward in a diabetic coma. This time he was very close to death, but once again medical expertise saved his life. The emergency ward doctor was puzzled. Yes, Marty had a severe diabetic condition, but insulin and strict adherence to a diet should have kept him in good shape. Could it be that his overall physical condition was deteriorating, or that the diabetes was becoming even more severe? These questions had been asked before, by the other doctors, and the answer had always been that the diabetes was *not* worse, nor was Marty's overall health. But now, once Marty was out of danger, this new doctor had a long talk with him. And Marty found it possible to respond, to talk about himself and the difficult life he was leading—to say things that had been bottled up for a long time, that he had never told anyone before. It was the right time—his life had just been saved, and he was grateful. The doctor was right too—he didn't act like a machine, he was a sincere guy.

What came out in that long talk and several others that followed? Marty had been diabetic for three years and had been in and out of hospitals innumerable times for examinations, laboratory studies, and treatment. An underweight, sickly, only child, he lived in the slums with his parents, who wanted him to be somebody—but they were split on how that would happen. Though Marty was bright in school, he was often in trouble—reprimanded, suspended, kicked out, reinstated. Even so, he had managed to reach senior year in high school, and his parents were hoping he would get to college. Marty didn't follow classmates who were involved in crime or in drugs, but he did get entangled in "causes." His conservative mother tried to make him a conformist. She didn't want him to become a revolutionary, she said, just a law-abiding, sensible citizen. They argued all the time about eating, his radical friends, girls, clothes, everything. The more she insisted on her views, the more irked and rebellious he got. His quiet father, who barely eked out a living, sided with him, encouraging him to think for himself, but he was no match for the vocal mother. When Marty was seventeen, he was bounced from high school for being involved in a student strike. There had been a terrible scene that evening; his parents had been very upset, and long after he had gone to bed he heard them arguing, his father defending him as usual. Suddenly there was a terrible scream. He ran into the kitchen and saw his father on the floor paralyzed, unable to talk, saliva running down his chin.

Though his father subsequently recovered from the stroke, Marty continued to feel terribly remorseful—as though he were to blame—until he was reinstated in school. That made his parents happy. Then the oppressive feelings of guilt toward his father subsided and finally seemed to have disappeared. He didn't know that a guilt which suddenly disappears from awareness without really being relieved signals the strong possibility of impending body disturbance, and that he would be paying with his body for something that had been erased from his conscious mind. The price was his first diabetic coma.

His antagonism toward his mother increased; the more she hovered over him, insisting on the insulin and the diet, the more he was impelled to neglect the insulin and flaunt the diet. He was expressing anger and rebellion through this behavior. The doctor who rescued him did more than regulate Marty's blood sugar. He gained Marty's trust, listened to his terrible emotional dilemma, and picked up the psychological signs that revealed how hard it was for Marty to follow his diet and take his insulin regularly. The doctor was able to make a few simple connections that gave Marty at least a start toward freeing himself from his hangups.

All of us should try to find a doctor who will be interested not only in our bodily ailments but also in the emotional signals that reveal how complicated the course of our illness may become.

PREDICTING REACTIONS TO PHYSICAL EXAMINATION

Emotions may influence our reactions to even a routine physical examination. For instance, Barry, a middle-aged bachelor, who had postponed having a checkup for several years, began to feel tense when he finally went to his doctor, especially when he was told his prostate gland was about to be examined. As the doctor's rubber-gloved finger entered his anus, Barry fainted. It was a response to sudden, intense anxiety. Later, when he had recovered, he admitted that he felt rather sheepish over what had happened, and that this very procedure had been on his mind from the time he had made the appointment for his checkup. It had been a sign that something untoward might happen during the examination. He had, however, denied his concern so well that he was unaware of his true feelings until the last moment.

As a youngster and during adolescence Barry had some-times tried anal stimulation while masturbating, but this had made him feel so dirty he finally had given it up. However, the desire to do this remained, though it was outside his awareness and dormant for a long time. Some months before his physical examination, a male colleague at work tried to seduce him, and Barry had rejected his advances indignantly. But this stirred up old fantasies, and Barry reacted to the rectal examination as if it had a sexual meaning. Most men respond to the doctor's examining finger with only mild spasm and general uneasiness which quickly passes.

Similarly, some women react to a vaginal examination as if it were a highly sexualized procedure. Consider Miss

Jenny, a timid, inhibited person in her late thirties. Her one affair with a man had been very brief and without physical pleasure. Though she was no longer a virgin, every time she visited her doctor it was a big defensive production because she immediately had fantasies of rape and assault. These were signs that the examination would be difficult, but she did not reveal them. Her internist was a kindly, fatherly man, but Miss Jenny enveloped herself in sheets, shuddered at any exposure of her naked body, and was not at all reassured by the presence of the nurse. In her case, this fear of men went back to childhood. She had had a loud, bossy father who had frequently beaten her. She remembered her mother as always whimpering, reduced to a meaningless role in the family. As Miss Jenny grew up, all men became fused in her thinking with her father's image. All men were suspect.

MORE ABOUT OVERREACTING TO TREATMENT

A few more words about treatment. If the clues suggesting that you will overreact to treatment are ignored and you are inadequately prepared for it emotionally, you may become terribly anxious or may feel that you are giving in and had no choice. Then your tension and resentment, if blocked from direct expression, will come out in the form of depression or apathy, or—which is the most undesirable—may be a factor in puzzling slowness of recovery. If you are inclined to be sensitive and not to take orders easily, crude pressure may result in your outright refusal to follow medical advice; you may even leave the hospital and the doctor.

Your emotional reactions to clinical and laboratory procedures are determined by many factors. Your illness itself —any pain, fever, or discomfort—will have a bearing; so will your mental attitude (whether fearful or optimistic), your trust or distrust of your doctors and nurses, the particular symbolic meaning a given procedure may have for you, and your previous experiences with hospitals or bouts of illness at home. All of these factors are present in all of us, but their relative importance will differ from one individual to another. Unfortunately, most of us are slow to grasp that it is not just the ailment itself, but also the emotions it arouses in us, which signal suffering, complications, prolonged recovery, or even relapse.

Of course, I'm not saying that our emotions always cause us to delay seeing our doctors or reject or resist medical advice. But they are involved much more often than we suspect.

It is all-important to remember that there are signs that foretell whether we will distort the perceptions of our bodies, and that predict our reactions to bodily ailments and to those who minister to us. The more these are known and understood, the more prepared we and our physician will be to deal effectively with the many complications that ill health can bring into our lives.

18

Before and After Surgery

Many lives have been saved by skillful surgery. Over twelve million operations a year are performed in the United States. Diseased bodily parts are removed, injuries repaired, deformities corrected, and organs transplanted. But what about people who die after an operation, or who remain sick when an uneventful convalescence was anticipated, or who have complications that don't respond to the best medical and surgical efforts? That emotion plays a role in the recovery process seems indisputable. Yet some surgeons dismiss emotion as irrelevant, not only in their patients, but in themselves. Surgical skill and technique are their principal interests. The operation's the thing. But there are psychological clues about the outcome of an operation which, if heeded, will either prevent or lessen unfavorable results. Naturally it would be absurd to expect your surgeon to analyze your feelings. But it's not at all unreasonable of you to expect him to have *some* understanding of you as a person, to recognize when you have hangups, and if necessary, get you expert help for them. However, your expectations may not be realized. So some knowledge of emotional reactions that occur before and after surgery—and the signals they transmit concerning the course of the illness—could be useful to you or your relatives and close friends. Let's begin with the more extreme responses.

PREOPERATIVE PSYCHOLOGICAL SIGNALS

Certain people are extremely upset by the prospect of surgery but totally deny their concern. This may be a sign that they will have a postoperative psychosis. Paradoxically, a few who *are* psychotic but must be operated on may show extraordinary mental improvement afterward. Then there are others who are always looking for a surgical solution for their symptoms. This surgical enthusiasm can be foreseen in their insatiable desire to be cared for, even if it means being cut first; or there may be an urgent need to be relieved of tormenting guilt, so that the operation is seen (irrationally) as punishment. In such people, conflicts can lead to physical symptoms which so mimic a surgical condition that many a surgeon will be convinced that an operation is indicated. Usually little or no physical disease is found. Unfortunately, such people are probably more familiar to the surgeon than to the psychiatrist.

A dramatic example is a woman who at age twenty-one already had been able to get twenty-eight operations done on different parts of her body. She was unusual, but less striking instances of such addiction are not uncommon. Most surgeons shy away from the much-operated patient, recognizing that something has gone awry in these people. There are, however, a few doctors who will operate just once more.

Suppose that something is amiss with your body and you begin to think, rightly or wrongly, that you're going to need an operation. Quite likely the worst possibilities will pass through your mind—if not a fatal outcome, then some crippling deformity or an ugly scar. Or you think of being anesthetized, unconscious, and never waking up again. Excessive anxiety is a signal that you will probably delay consulting a doctor. As in other instances of illness already discussed, such delay can mean unnecessary suffering, since you may be mistaken about your condition and not require surgery at all. Should you need an operation, then continuing, unrelieved, severe tension usually assures that there will be complications—*physical* as well as mental. So expecting the worst is an attitude we should try to avoid, although often we'll need help to do this.

On the other hand, some of us seem utterly indifferent to our bodies, and deny or make light of symptoms unrealistically. That, too, is a sign that we may be diverted into the trap of waiting, waiting when we have a progressively worsening physical condition—until surgery comes too late, or almost too late. This extreme form of indifference is a variation of a healthier attitude known as *minimization*. This attitude is a psychological defense that may serve us in good stead while we are waiting to be taken to the operating room. Thus minimization is an attempt, as its name implies, to lessen the seriousness of what lies ahead. It is an attempt to adapt, to spare ourselves too great anxiety by concentrating on the optimistic side of things. Only when it is carried to the extreme does it become unhealthy.

Here is an example. A patient is scheduled for reconstructive surgery involving the tear ducts. He is calm, cool, and affable. This absence of any tension whatsoever is noted by his surgeon who, however, gives it no further thought. The operation is started under local anesthesia. For the first fifteen minutes all goes well. Then the patient's heart suddenly stops beating. Immediate emergency measures are instituted. The heartbeat starts up again before any critical interval has elapsed.

Later a nurse, in the course of talking with the patient, learns that while having an impacted molar extracted six months previously, he had fainted in the middle of the procedure. The patient is a high-level executive who never lost his cool, even in the past year when he was in charge of a number of labor disputes in his company. But bottled-up emotions now have twice made their impact felt on his body.

OVERANXIOUS PARENTS

Sometimes, when surgery has been recommended, the emotional trauma it is expected to cause is exaggerated. How can we tell this? Suppose that you're the psychologically sophisticated but overanxious parent of a child facing an operation. You find it hard to give your consent, because you think the child's stability will be irreparably damaged. You concentrate on the symbolic meaning of the operation (often what it means to *you*—not to your child!) and underestimate your child's ability to adapt to stress. You also forget, or don't take sufficiently into account, that the stress of an operation can often be reduced or neutralized by such measures as adequate emotional preparation of the child; or the possibility of the mother's living-in (allowed in some hospitals, but not advised for emotionally unstable mothers, whose presence would upset the child all the more); or the provision for substitute mothering in addition to regular medical and nursing care—which would cushion the impact of separation from parents (some hospitals have special staff for this purpose). Let's consider a few actual cases.

Mark, age four, a rather anxious child, had very large adenoids which interfered with his breathing. His snore at night was truly impressive. His parents, both steeped in psychological lore, had been advised that the adenoids should come out. But they could not reach a decision to go ahead. They were afraid the operation and separation from his parents might create such a strain for Mark that he would never get over it. Finally they went to see a psychiatric consultant about their dilemma. He recognized the nature of the impasse and advised that they get another opinion from a topnotch surgeon and follow it. If surgery was recommended, Mark could be prepared emotionally for it and arrangements made for the mother to stay with him after the operation. When he awoke from the anesthesia, he would see her familiar face. Then, under the guidance of the nursing staff, she could assist with his care overnight. What actually happened? The need for the operation was confirmed, the child was properly prepared, and the suggested hospital arrangements were made. The parents felt considerably relieved, and Mark went through surgery without ill effect.

In another instance, the parents—also psychologically sophisticated—were very troubled when their first baby was born with a cleft palate. They were told that surgical intervention at the age of eighteen months would cure the condition. The parents were informed that in this particular hospital, it was policy that the child not be seen by them for a week after the operation. The explanation: when they left after each visit, the child would cry, the sutures would not remain in place, and the cleft would open up again. The parents were so concerned about the effect the long separation would have on the child that they panicked. The surgeon did not understand what was causing their indecision. But when they were informed by another doctor and saw for themselves that warm and sympathetic mothering care was indeed available and given to the little patients on the surgical ward, the parents felt considerably reassured. Overanxious parents also can be helped by learning in advance how to deal with their feelings about the hospitalized child, even when he's getting good care.

ADAPTIVE RESPONSES

However, no one, child or adult, is happy at the prospect of going under the knife. Patient to surgeon: "I'm not a hero—I'm afraid of having an operation." Surgeon to patient: "You're not a hero, but you're an honest man. No real heroes enter the operating room." Almost always surgery looms as a threat. And we, as adults, deal with this threat in many different ways—each a sign of how we are trying to adjust.

One of my patients, awaiting removal of an ovarian cyst, had vivid fantasies that she was a cavalry officer, riding a spirited horse and swiping away at fleeing men with a great sword. This was a way of relieving the strain she was under; she imagined that she was in command, so neither the surgeon nor the operation could hurt her. She had had similar fantasies in childhood each time she had been beaten by her brutal, alcoholic father. They were of some help then and also now in her attempts to adapt to cruel reality. She was identifying with the aggressor.

Another patient, fearful of being helpless and at the mercy of the surgeon, protected himself by being as uncooperative as he could. For instance, as part of the preoperative preparation he was given an enema, but he retained it to such an extent that it was absorbed in his bowel, and as a result, *nothing* came out. He said this reminded him of his childhood, when he stubbornly held back bowel movements despite pleading, cajoling, and even threats from his mother. In this case, the patient's emotional conditioning did not help, but worked against him. He resisted anesthesia, and postoperatively he was plagued by constipation.

Still another patient awaiting surgery invented elaborate explanations as to why he was upset, but he blamed it all on some business affairs which actually turned out to be trivial. In other words, to avoid anxiety about the operation, he became concerned about totally unrelated matters. The shift was not effective in helping him cope with his tension, which remained at a high level. A stubborn wound infection marred his convalescence for weeks.

CHILDHOOD CONDITIONING

Even if you try to approach surgery in a relatively calm and objective fashion, you'll still find anxious thoughts and feelings sneaking into your mind. Many of these fears will probably be childhood ones that have become stirred up by the current stress of waiting for surgery. The extent to which childhood experience enters into such a situation varies enormously from one person to the next. But most of us will feel some degree—probably too great and unrealistic a degree—of helplessness. Going to the hospital may activate old fears of abandonment by those close to us. Or we may have elaborate fantasies of being subjected to punishment for some wrong we have imagined or done. If you are a man, preoccupation with thoughts of being cut by the surgeon's scalpel may stir up long-submerged fears of losing your genitals because you had forbidden sexual fantasies and activities. It's common for little boys to imagine that their father will wield a knife against them to put an end to "dirty" thinking and behavior. So for men, surgery may symbolize castration, even though the actual operation is in a body area away from the sex organs. If you are a woman, the surgeon's activities may symbolically represent rape or mutilation. Again, unpleasant childhood memories or fantasies of a cruel parent or some overbearing and brutal adult have been stirred up.

Operations in childhood can leave a special and disturbing imprint on your subsequent emotional life, if they have been done without any regard for the state of your feelings at the time. Then, under such circumstances, anesthesia and surgery tend to become fearfully distorted. They activate feelings of helplessness and expectations of abandonment, mutilation, even annihilation. These are signals that children facing surgery while their parents are away will have an especially stormy time of it. For example, a youngster, although cared for by a well-trained governess, missed his mother very much while she was on a European trip. The only sign of this was his frenetic overactivity. During this time he "accidentally" broke his leg, which required surgical intervention under a general anesthetic, and which took an awfully long time to heal. He remained moody and irritable for many months afterward, even when his mother returned.

For him this highly traumatic (physical as well as emotional) event symbolized a final separation from mother and possibly from life itself. When, as an adult, he was operated on for an overactive thyroid gland, the loneliness and anger associated with his earlier hospitalization came back to him, and his recovery again took a long time. Irrespective of age, sophistication, or education, all patients (even doctors!) who face major surgery regress to some extent. Sometimes the more uninformed you are about what to expect, the more severe the regression is apt to be. Long-buried childish fears linked with fantasy and actual experience are activated and mingle with mature thoughts and attitudes.

THE TENSION OF OTHERS

Another sign that points to complications in surgery is the presence in the sickroom of long-faced family and friends. Their verbal and nonverbal communication with you, the patient, will be loaded with anxiety and depression. Your own attitudes can then be affected unfavorably and, in turn, your body. Even more disturbing to you will be a tense anesthetist or surgeon. Your confidence level will plummet, and your anxiety level will skyrocket. Suppose, though, instead of responding with alarm, you become very quiet, seemingly showing no emotion. Actually you may be paralyzed by fear. Marked, overt anxiety or the opposite—lying in bed "dead-still"—are extremes of emotional response that foretell trouble during and after surgery.

SPECIFIC OPERATIONS, SPECIFIC ANXIETIES

The kind of operation you're going to have will affect, to some extent, the content of your anxious thinking about what lies ahead. For instance, brain surgery is associated with subsequent mental disturbance; an eye operation, with blindness; chest and heart, with sudden death; urinary tract in males, impotence; reproductive system in women, loss of femininity; bones, interference with mobility. The more minor an operation, the greater the concern associated with anesthesia, whereas major operations evoke more anxiety about the outcome of the surgery.

So what is being done to counter the unpleasant emotions that all of us experience before surgery? It is true that in modern (and often the most expensive) hospitals, the operating rooms, recovery rooms, and patients' rooms are being redesigned to be more pleasant and functional. You may even have modulated stereo music softly playing as you are anesthetized. Then you are wheeled into the sterile operating room with controlled ventilation and bacteria-repellent walls. Technically, every precaution will be taken to ensure a germ-free, soundproof atmosphere, but recognition of your emotional needs cannot be built into hospital architecture. Whether you are to have a general anesthetic—used for the vast majority of operations—so that you will not know what's going on during the operation, or whether you will be conscious under regional or spinal anesthesia, or nerve block, in any case a kindly face or voice, a few reassuring words from nurses, anesthetist, and surgeon before surgery will make a great deal of difference.

POSTOPERATIVE PSYCHOLOGICAL SIGNS

When your operation is over and you are in the recovery room or intensive care unit and later in your room, it takes a while for things to get into focus as the anesthetic wears off. Meanwhile relatives and friends are tensely awaiting word of how things went. How both you and those close to you are handled varies considerably from hospital to hospital. Despite inevitable emergencies and lack of personnel, it seems reasonable to expect a few words from the surgeon to calm your relatives, and some arrangement so that your return to consciousness may be in the presence of a reassuring voice and a kindly face. Certainly, if your surgeon suspects an untoward physical reaction to the operation, he will take great care to keep you under constant surveillance. But if you also need emotional support as you reorient yourself, what will be ordered for you, or what will be available then? It is true that some patients come out of anesthesia with little difficulty and display a quick ability to cooperate and help themselves even while still in the recovery room. Their convalescence is apt to be free of complications. But others come out of anesthesia very slowly, and their readjustment to reality is quite painful. These are signs that much support will be necessary in the postoperative period.

As time passes after the operation, you will continue to react not only physically but also in psychological ways. If there are no immediate physical complications, your first reaction will probably be great relief, then elation. You may feel as if you have returned from the dead. But that state of mind may not last long. You may be troubled by pain, various disturbances of bodily functions, inability to move freely, or awareness that a bodily part has been removed. It is normal then to find yourself irritable and depressed. But if these emotional indicators persist, are not recognized, and the upheaval behind them is not worked through to some extent, that in turn is a sign that convalescence may become complicated and drawn out.

EMOTIONAL RESPONSE TO AMPUTATION

It used to be that, if you lost a limb, you might be haunted for a long time afterward by the illusion that the limb was still there, by persistent pain coming from that area, and by a terrible feeling of inferiority. In the most extreme cases, you might be kept from leading a useful life; the loss could have a paralyzing effect on your body and mind. Preoperatively, this is signaled when you show extraordinary concern about any alteration in the integrity of your body image. Fortunately some surgeons are beginning to recognize these signals, and to include their patients' emotions as well as their bodies in the treatment.

For example of such an enlightened and comprehensive approach, consider Brendan, who had been a fireman for twenty-five years and had more than a few scars to show for the lieutenant's badge he now wore. The night his company responded to a three-bagger in an abondoned warehouse, Brendan felt in his bones that he would be unlucky. It was a stubborn fire. While he was directing his men near a particularly hot spot in the blazing building, a wall suddenly gave way. A heavy slab of masonry landed on Brendan's leg, crushing it beyond repair. The terrible pain was dulled by a shot of morphine, so Brendan at first didn't realize what was going to happen to him when he got to the hospital. Just before the anesthetic knocked him out, he was briefly aware of terror. The leg was amputated above the knee. A few years ago Brendan would have awakened to the emotional shock of amputation, with his first postoperative impressions focused wholly on his loss. But he was lucky because his surgeon did something unusual. He attached a temporary artificial limb right after the operation, while Brendan was still under anesthesia. When he awoke, his first impression was not "A part of me is gone, lost forever." Instead, some sense of intactness was preserved in him. The effect on Brendan's morale, on his emotional balance, was a softening of the cruel blow, so that his recovery was swifter.

After an operation you will be aware of unpleasant sensations and feelings, or be wrapped in hazy consciousness or dulled pain. It is a time for your nurses and doctors to be on the lookout not only for physical complications but for psychological signs that recovery will be slowed up. The latter indications will be even more clearly evident if your visitors—family and friends—upset you. But such telltale signs will be missed if your doctors and nurses are impervious to anything but the condition of your body. What does one look for? Are you reacting too passively, almost infant-like, to your condition? Are you overly fearful and tearful? Are you inappropriately angry, refusing the most simple procedures, such as having your temperature or blood pressure taken?

PSYCHOLOGICAL FORECASTING IN TRANSPLANTATION

All of these clues—although common in ordinary surgery—are present in more complex form in the case of some of the newer and stranger surgical techniques, such as kidney transplants. You will have undergone a complicated operation and many physical procedures before and after. Your emotional reactions will be very special. Here are some indications of the presence of tension potentially harmful to your body, and especially to the transplant.

If you are not one of those people who deny their feelings, you may first have a fantasy that you're harboring something foreign and fragile, something that's sticking out. It may take a while to get used to the transplant, to think of it as part of yourself, and finally to be no longer aware of it. But then, if something has to be done to it, you may again perceive it anxiously as something that doesn't really belong to you. Suppose that your older brother donated the kidney. A part of him is inside you. You are urinating with his kidney. This reinforcement of identification with him may be accompanied by the adoption of some other traits of his, such as his mannerisms, posture, way of walking. And guilt may trouble you. Will his life be shortened by what he's done for you? This concern becomes very great if he should become ill. You may fear not only that it is your fault if something terrible happens to him, but you may also fear that his illness will be reflected in the kidney he donated to you. In other words, in your mind you could well imagine that you and your brother are now inseparable Siamese twins.

Children who are recipients of kidney transplants are faced with special emotional burdens that may jeopardize the continuation of their newly found health. They who have been so sick now return home much revitalized but changed in appearance and slowed in growth. The process of becoming reintegrated into the family fold is a complicated one and the source of further indications of how recovery will go. Is the child able to get used to his bodily changes, forget hospital living, and readjust to his parents and siblings, who may have strained feelings toward him because of his illness? Is going back to school especially stressful? Parents may even fall into the awful trap of using the transplant to control the child's behavior. Suppose the parent is the donor and then threatens: "If you do that naughty thing again, I'll take back my kidney" or "You'd better take care of my kidney or you'll lose it." The consequences will be terrible, both emotionally and physically.

And overhanging all recipients of organ transplants is the fear of short life expectancy, even though several years have gone by since the operation. How can the many pitfalls be avoided, the upsets lessened? In these especially difficult cases of transplants (including the more recent work with heart transplantation), the psychological signs are especially important in alerting doctors, nurses, social workers, family, and friends to the patient's great need for support and understanding both before and after the operation. Sensitive and skillful professional counseling—preferably, in most instances, psychotherapy—is called for. In the case of kidney transplantation, this is true not only for the recipient, but also for the donor—especially if the donor is a relative or otherwise in close contact with the patient.

RECOVERY—MORE APPARENT THAN REAL

That emotional problems accompany transplants may seem obvious, since we don't yet look on transplants as an everyday type of surgery. But many, many emotional problems also accompany the less exotic surgical procedures that are done by the millions every year. If your physical progress following surgery seems to be good, your psychological state will probably be disregarded by your surgeon, unless your emotions get so out of hand that you show signs of becoming psychotic. If you've *physically* recovered from the operation, you are considered to be *totally* recovered. Yet sometimes, after leaving the hospital, you may become mysteriously anxious and depressed. Sometimes, too, you develop physical symptoms. Is that because some new illness has developed? In my opinion the more likely explanation is that your original illness had been triggered by an activated emotional conflict; now that surgery has "corrected" the first way your body responded to that psychological upset, your body has found a new way to react, a new illness. That's because the original triggering emotions have not been sufficiently deactivated.

For instance, in the hospital where I was on the staff, an elevator operator had spoken to me briefly about his troubles. He was thirty-five years old, living unhappily with his parents, and subject to stomach upsets. A few days before, he had had a terrible argument with them which had left him feeling drained of emotion—or so he described it. But although he was unaware of it, his fury at them and himself was evident to me. I suggested that he talk things over with his doctor. Some weeks later I learned he had been operated on for acute appendicitis. On his return to work,

223

when I asked him how he was, he said, "No more stomach trouble, Doc. But boy, have I been getting severe headaches!" His home situation and his difficult relationships with his parents had remained unchanged. He no longer had an appendix, but the impact of his still active conflicts had shifted to a new target organ in his body.

OPERATIONS THAT RELIEVE GUILT

Things don't always work out this way, though. Sometimes an operation has a symbolic meaning of atonement, thereby relieving the patient's bad conscience, and there are no complications—physical or emotional—for an indefinite period afterward. A young married woman had been harboring intense guilt over an affair she had had with another man just before she met her husband. Within a few months after beginning treatment with me, she developed an excruciating backache after lifting a heavy bundle of laundry at home. The pain grew worse, with radiation down her right leg. A diagnosis of slipped (intervertebral) disk was confirmed by special X ray. All treatment failed to give relief, and she could not walk. An operation was performed and the physical condition corrected. Her convalescence was uneventful. She felt better emotionally than she had in years. After a few more interviews she discontinued psychotherapy. Her emotional conflicts had not been resolved, but they had stopped troubling her. What she had gone through in surgery had relieved her guilt feelings as well as her slipped disk.

ANTICIPATING THE OUTCOME OF ELECTIVE SURGERY

A rather complicated case was Mrs. Prescott, who had always been high-strung. Now in her early forties, the mother of two rebellious adolescents, and married to a passive man who was going nowhere, she became increasingly upset. Her whole body felt irritated and tense. Her periods, usually uncomfortable, became irregular, painful, and profusely bloody. A finicky eater since childhood who always went off her feed and reacted with her stomach when anything happened, she picked at her food more than ever and complained of sour taste in her mouth, indigestion, and gas. Her doctor suggested that she was very nervous, but she argued she wasn't more nervous than anyone else. Then, after her mother, with whom she had never gotten along, died of cancer of the cervix which had spread throughout the body, she consulted the surgeon who had treated her mother. After a careful examination he could find no evidence of cancer. But he asked her to consider having her uterus removed. The pain, discomfort, and hemorrhaging would be over with, she already had children, and it would not interfere with her sexual life, which was nonexistent anyway because she had never experienced orgasm.

The surgeon assured her there was no emergency and the operation was entirely elective. A tricky word—elective. It generally refers only to the physical aspects of the condition and disregards altogether the patient's emotions, which could influence the decision, and the psychological indications of how surgery and convalescence would go. Mrs. Prescott, feeling strangely calm, decided to have her uterus out. The operation was routine, and then a varicose vein in her leg became inflamed and a blood clot found its way to her lungs, causing a serious pulmonary complication. She almost died.

Neither she nor her surgeon was aware that dangerous emotional conflicts had reached a critical point in her and that these foretold a possibly complicated recovery. Long before her operation she had been troubled by her poor relationship with her mother, and it had been a blow to have her mother die before they could come to terms. An extraordinary physical identification with her mother had taken place—not unusual in such cases—so that she developed similar symptoms even though she had no cancer. In a way, it was an attempt to find that elusive and longed-for union with her mother, but of course this identification was a very poor substitute for her loss and did nothing to assuage her guilt. The emotions that had been seething beneath the surface struck her body with full fury after the operation, and she was almost done in.

It took Mrs. Prescott the whole summer to recover. A year went by. No more periods and no more bleeding. But gas and indigestion continued to bother her. And she and her children and husband continued to be at loggerheads. Finally the children fled to colleges thousands of miles away. That upset her. Her ailing father paid her a brief visit. That upset her. When her family doctor, who had known her since childhood, again reminded her of her lifelong tendency to react with her stomach when anything upset her, she shrugged off his explanation as she had done so many times before.

As her symptoms recurred more frequently, she made a number of visits to different consultants, who varied in their opinions: nerves (she rejected psychotherapy); spastic colon (she tried tranquilizers, with little change); a beginning ulcer (the stomach X ray was ambiguous and the prescriptions did no good). Finally, the fourth expert ordered X rays of the gallbladder and found several small stones. After a long talk about possible chronic inflammation of the gallbladder and the likelihood that its removal would relieve her symptoms, Mrs. Prescott was again confronted with the decision—to be operated on or not to be operated on. Again it was elective. She thought of all the misery from her indigestion, gas, diarrhea, constipation, pain—and then about how the last operation had had unexpected complications—and finally decided she could live through this operation too. But this time she was apprehensive, aware of her anxiety. Her troubled emotions were more on the surface. Though no conflicts were resolved, the pent-up tensions found at least some release. And that may have been a contributing factor to why the surgery went without a hitch and the convalescence was uneventful. In a relatively short time she was up and about, though feeling somewhat weak and shaky. Had her emotional conflicts disappeared? No. She continued to be almost as upset as before, but she no longer had a gallbladder (or uterus). What organ would go next?

WHEN IS PLASTIC SURGERY CONTRAINDICATED?

Yes, surgery has many meanings for those who await it and for those who endure it. But one of the most extraordinary attitudes toward it is the expectation that it will rejuvenate us, fight off the ravages of time, give us a beautiful new appearance. Some people concerned with how they look, preoccupied with their faces, turn to surgery with hope that it will make their fondest fantasies come true. Vanessa was not an actress, not a model. She was a housewife who had been very attractive in her younger days—that is, to men other than her husband. He had never been interested in anything but his business. Vanessa had had a few discreet short-lived affairs, but not for some years now. Men weren't looking at her the way they used to. Her boredom grew. She took some courses at the university and lessons at a dance studio, and met a few handsome young men. She wanted sex and got only talk; they treated her like Mom. Mirrors in her home began to get a lot of use. She would stare at her face and neck for hours, counting the wrinkles, the bags beginning under her eyes, the skin sagging a little here and there. No longer a beauty, but still attractive for her age, she was discontented. She wanted to be young again, and all her thoughts and actions were directed toward that end: clothes, exercise, creams, visits to the beauty parlor, associating with young men. Finally she wound up in the office of the best plastic surgeon in town. She was stunned when he refused to operate. He said she was really searching for something that he couldn't give her—a sense of being somebody, a sense of belonging, a sense of peace with herself. What he did give her was the name of someone who dealt with these problems in other ways, a psychiatrist. And that's how Vanessa began somewhat late in her life to try to understand herself better.

The astute plastic surgeon has plenty of opportunity to note that results gratifying to his patients are achieved as much through psychological factors as through technical skills. This specialist will be cautious about correcting some slight defect or promising cosmetic changes when it is clear that the prospective patient hopes for something far greater—frequently the overcoming of intense inferiority feelings—and attaches too much importance to the outcome. Many people have plastic surgery that is technically successful, but are as discontented as ever because their neurotic expectations aren't met. Conversely, other people have so much faith in the surgeon that even though the operation does not turn out too well cosmetically, they are delighted with the results because some psychological need to achieve a new image has been satisfied by the surgeon's ministrations. Emotional factors and what they signal are especially complicated and should be taken into consideration whenever plastic surgery is contemplated.

USING PSYCHOLOGICAL SIGNS IN SURGERY

Whatever the reason for an operation—to save life or for cosmetic effect—it is done not just on a body but on a human being with feelings. All of us, without exception, whether awaiting surgery, undergoing it, or convalescing from it, will react emotionally. And our reactions will manifest themselves in many different ways, sometimes hidden, sometimes openly dramatic. These reactions indicate whether physical complications are in the offing.

What can be done before the operation? We need preparation, and not just physical preparation. We will be tense, waiting for the knife. A simple, reassuring outline of what lies ahead will have a steadying effect on us and give us a frame of reference instead of leaving us in apprehensive ignorance. We don't need any lecture on anatomy or pathology—but an understandable description of the procedures before the operation and those that most likely will be necessary afterward. And we also need a chance to talk about our fears and ask the questions that trouble us about the operation and its aftermath. Kindly human contact is more important than architecture in a hospital, especially when we are facing surgery. Even if the surgeon is busy and harassed, time spent talking with us in a comforting and sympathetic (but not syrupy or forced) way will lessen the possibility of later complications related to emotional upset.

It is not only the doctor, but the nurse and others, including warm-hearted paraprofessionals, who can provide the support that is so helpful before surgery. Only in acute emergencies will there be little opportunity to do this. But what's been outlined is really only minimum psychological preparation. If the specific emotional indications already described are looked for, additional knowledge can be gained about whether complications are likely. Then preventive measures can be taken, that is, the patient can be built up psychologically, in addition to being prepared physically for the shock of the operation.

When the surgeon is operating at his best, he is coolly objective, focused on your physical condition, and not disturbed by emotional distraction from within or without. And

229

that's the way it should be. Suppose, though, you are not under a general anesthetic. The complete surgeon will make a quick survey of your emotional state, again looking for signs of trouble. Are you panicky, extremely tense? Are you utterly impassive, without feeling? This indicates that some quick intervention would be in order. Calm, reassuring words from the surgeon may do much to lessen your natural as well as neurotic tension on the operating table. And such intervention need not interfere with the doctor's concentration.

And after the operation? Reorientation to the world as the anesthetic wears off is slow and gradual for us. Kindly human contact is essential from the surgeon, other doctors, nurses, social workers, dieticians, physiotherapists, and all who have anything to do with patients.

Seemingly strange behavior by patients and complications or slowness of recovery need careful exploration, not only from the physical standpoint. Are there emotional signs, not necessarily of a dramatic or overt kind, involved—grief over loss of a part of the body, depression over separation from family, activation of painful memories, undue hostility toward doctors and nurses, suspiciousness, apprehension over the future? Or apathy, listlessness, lack of interest in what's going on around you, confusion? Operations have hidden meanings for us. These needn't necessarily be understood in depth, but the signs just mentioned are specific warnings of a stormy convalescence. Surgical success has to be measured not just by physical recovery from the specific ailment, but also in terms of our subsequent health. Operations may settle down a raging emotional conflict—or not. If the former occurs, better health lies ahead. If the latter, then our difficulties will continue or quickly return, either in emotional or physical form.

Very recently, surgical and psychological know-how (strange bedfellows) have joined together to prevent some postoperative complications, such as phantom-leg pain following amputation, described earlier. You are not treated as a machine with a defective part that has to be replaced, but as a *person* in distress. This combination of surgical and psychological expertise is being extended to the process of rehabilitation in which morale and will to recover combine to play important roles. It is hoped that technical surgical skills and knowledge of human nature will *both* continue to be applied more and more in surgery—before, during, and after the operation.

19

Forever Sick

WORK, ACCIDENTS, AND PENSIONS

It was Rocky's first accident in twenty years. In all that time as a construction worker, he had weathered many tough jobs without a scratch. Skill and luck had probably been the reasons. Now a sudden gust of wind tipped a pile of bricks on the new skyscraper scaffolding and sent them raining down. Rocky was on the ground level and heard the yells, but not soon enough. Had he become a little careless, or were his reflexes slowing down? Several bricks bounced off his helmet, tilting it, and another struck his unprotected head a glancing blow and knocked him out. Rocky was in the hospital a week with a bad brain concussion. When he returned home to convalesce, he couldn't get rid of the dizziness, and the headache hung on and on, despite all the medicines. Rocky was awarded disability compensation without question and given a long leave of absence from his job. His wife and kids had a hard time getting used to his new grouchiness. He was uncomfortable at home, but when he thought of going back to work, he would break out in a cold sweat and his heart would begin to pound. He also kept having nightmares of dodging big girders as they swung all around him and would wake up screaming, scaring his wife out of her wits. He couldn't return to work; his explanation made sense to him and to everyone he knew—he had real headaches and dizziness, and they didn't get any better.

No one expected a man subject to so much suffering to go back to work.

What really held him back was anxiety, a loss of confidence in himself. But he couldn't admit that. No one knew, although perhaps his wife guessed some nervous change had taken place in him. Being ill or injured can do that to us—make us lose confidence, so that we feel very discouraged about again being independent and must rely on others for support. Even if such support seems to be simply financial compensation for physical injury and illness—either in the form of disability or pension payments—it usually means more than money. It's also a symbol of being looked after, and it doesn't matter if it's the union, the company, or the state—what matters is that *someone* is looking after us again, just as our parents used to do when we were kids and could not assume responsibilities on our own. A little of that need to be cared for is in all of us. But in some of us there's a lot of it. In some of us the craving for reassurance, attention, comfort, and pity can become exaggerated—especially if we are disabled. Then our feelings of helplessness and insecurity increase that need even more. And if the injury or sickness brings all the attention we ever wanted, it'll be hard to get well. We probably won't see it this way—like Rocky, we'll find lots of "valid" reasons for remaining dependent on others—but our basic problem will be our unwillingness to give up a good thing. Unconsciously or unwittingly, we keep ourselves ill, to ensure that these emotional (as well as financial) goodies keep coming.

So, strange as it may seem, disease or injury can be extremely satisfying and rewarding. In fact, to find satisfaction in illness is so common that it even has a name—*secondary gain*. It is a prime psychological sign that a disability will linger on indefinitely. It's not difficult to come under the spell of secondary gain. The effect of our symptoms on our employer, on the law, and on our family and friends can be highly dramatic, especially if our disability casts us in the role of a hero—even a martyr—for a while. Those around us will tend to make fewer demands on us (especially if *their* guilty feelings are stirred up), will be more solicitous and sympathetic, and may even give up their own pleasures to avoid upsetting us. Actually, many people who are chronically ill or seriously disabled learn to become quite adept at manipulating people around them and using them for selfish purposes. Undoubtedly all of us have had some experience with the tyranny of sick people—either ourselves or others—because it is such a common occurrence. We all tend to be somewhat demanding and self-centered when we are ill—some of us more than others. There is no harm in this so long as we use it to fulfill a small and temporary need for attention. But it can indeed become dangerous when we let it get out of hand and become a way of life. Then it works as a powerful motivation *against* our getting better and *for* living off others.

"I CAN'T LET GO OF HER"

Mrs. Howell had been a grande dame in her social set until her husband, a prominent banker, died suddenly. Then her own health began to decline and she was found to have diabetes and arteriosclerotic heart disease, both mild. From an outgoing, party-giving person she changed into a semi-invalid who rarely saw anyone any more. For many years Mrs. Howell had compensated, indeed overcompensated, for her basically shy, timid, and dependent personality by a façade which was just the opposite. Her husband, a gregarious, hard-working, and hard-drinking type, had really carried her along by sheer force of his own dynamic behavior. His sudden death had been a shocking blow. The emotional props on which she had relied for so many years had been taken from her forever. Preoccupation with death made her frequently moody and irritable. Although her physician placed little restriction on her activities, she chose to give up her former mode of existence. She sold the family mansion and settled with her spinster daughter Patsy into a fashionable apartment. Life with her daughter became increasingly strained, but Mrs. Howell was afraid to be alone: what if she had a heart attack and could not summon help? Besides, she needed Patsy's companionship. She had no confidence that anyone else would stay with her. When tensions between her and her daughter rose, the mother would complain of heart flutter and difficulty in breathing.

During each crisis the family physician came and found Mrs. Howell's pulse to be quite irregular; despite a bit of congestion in her lungs, it was not a life-threatening situation. But she could not rest easy, did not feel reassured, felt unable to follow her doctor's advice to mobilize herself, and even cheated a bit on the medication, insisting that the pills did no good anyway. After all, if she were ill, Patsy would *have* to be concerned. Mrs. Howell, constantly afraid Patsy might leave her, resented and thwarted any effort by her daughter to have a social life of her own. All Mrs. Howell would have to do was have a relapse. As Patsy approached an early menopause, her chances of getting married fading, she made an attempt at one last relationship, but her mother's physical condition immediately took a marked turn for the worse—or so it seemed. Patsy blamed herself for causing this setback in her mother's condition and gave up her lover. Through her sickness Mrs. Howell had made certain of her daughter's staying with her. Unfortunately, Patsy had established such a habit of responding to this pressure that it was impossible to free herself from her mother's emotional clutches.

RELIEVING YOUR CONSCIENCE

But tying others to us is only one way that we use secondary gain. Ill health, through the suffering it imposes, may relieve our own troubled conscience. This is a more subtle form of satisfaction from illness. Suppose that you, a married man, have been fooling around on the side, but find yourself feeling terribly guilty. You become noticeably depressed. Then your arthritis kicks up. Your ankles get swollen and terribly painful. The illness forces you into bed for a while, despite the best treatment. It's hard to sleep. You can hardly move your legs. Your wife is concerned. The boss tells you to take all the time off from work that you need. But more impressive than anything else is the fact you're no longer depressed. Despite the bodily discomfort, you feel a curious sense of relief. Nobody knows this but you, and you don't know why. But actually your physical suffering has relieved your mental suffering. This is a little-heard-of but not uncommon way of deriving some gain from an illness, and a sign that it will endure.

EXCUSES, EXCUSES

Many people use physical disability as an excuse for avoiding family or job responsibilities, for being unable to meet financial obligations, or for escaping from legal consequences. Consider how Willie reacted. He was back from the war in Vietnam with a Purple Heart, a right hand and arm that didn't seem to be much use to him, and a pension. The pain just wouldn't go away. When he was a kid, Willie had injured that arm pitching Little League baseball, a severe muscle strain had laid him up for several weeks, and his mother had fussed over him. In Vietnam he took shrapnel from an enemy ambush and got a messy wound which took quite a while to heal. He had little enthusiasm for the rehabilitation program set up to restore function in the wounded arm and hand. Here he was back in the States, but the damn ache came back with him. He had no drive and couldn't get going on work, or studies, or anything. Deep down Willie was very passive, and even before his wound had been terribly unsure of himself, but nobody knew about that. Everyone excused him because he had been severely wounded, so no one was expecting him to go anywhere. Even when he met *the* girl, she was most understanding and insisted that after they were married she would continue to work as long as necessary; with his pension they would get along until he was able to really stand on his own two feet. Willie saw this as proof of her love for him. She cared despite his physical incapacity. And so the years slipped by—and Willie's secondary gain, his avoidance of psychotherapy and other rehabilitative measures continued, and that arm and hand didn't get better. Such an outcome could have been predicted.

FORETELLING RESISTANCE TO RECOVERY

When illness excuses you from facing and dealing with unpleasant realities in your life, you may not even want to get better. Something in you will resist the best efforts to improve your physical condition. What are the indications that this might occur? They are often little things like misunderstanding simple directions, forgetting to take medicine, neglecting exercises, missing appointments for checkups, and doing what you've been told to avoid. If you have become accustomed to such forms of resistance, you will give them up only when the suffering from your illness becomes far greater than the emotional gains derived from it.

Some people who are receiving financial compensation

or other benefits from illness protest loudly that they would rather have their health; they can cast blame on all those associated with treating them, complaining that medical and nursing incompetence is the reason for their not getting well. Actually, in such instances, they are often simply trying to cover up for severe dependent needs that existed long before the illness. Possibly they were unaware of the dependency until the illness started, so it's easy for them to see all their problems as caused by the illness—and the doctors attending it—rather than the other way 'round.

SECONDARY GAIN IN CHILDHOOD

How we respond to illness or injury in childhood can give clues to how we will react later in life. As children we are quite open and frank about using a disability—even though it's minor—as a reason for escaping chores or staying home from school. The secondary gain is even greater when our illness or injury makes our parents give us too much attention and care, and parents often can become overanxious and overprotective when their own emotional problems make them see their sick child as an extension of themselves. Sometimes parents may even be oversolicitous because that's a way of concealing the fact that they really resent the child. In any event, as youngsters we may learn to take advantage of illness as a prime way of gaining attention, warding off punishment, and avoiding other unpleasant situations. Then, as adults, we may continue to use any bodily disorder to gain similar emotional ends.

In children, the discovery that injury may yield some pleasant returns can be used by them to adapt to situations that otherwise might be too painful and depressing. It becomes dangerous only when using a disability to gain some self-centered end is so well rewarded, works so successfully, that the child begins to make it a habit, a way of life. Take this five-year-old who hit his eye with a wooden block a day before the family was to leave for a week's vacation in ski country. The parents and older children could ski, but the patient couldn't; he felt he would be left out of the fun. Unfortunately, the doctor bungled the treatment —he thought the injury was a simple cut and just put a couple of stitches in the eyelid. But the child complained he could not see with that eye, so the parents took him to a consultant, who found that there had been some bleeding in it. The specialist didn't consider the condition serious, but both eyes had to be covered with patches and the child was immobilized in bed for five days.

The maternal grandmother offered to look after him, but the parents, overly anxious about the outcome, called off the vacation. The child was somewhat irritable and tense, and the parents, perhaps because they felt guilty about their annoyance at missing the vacation, spent a lot of time fussing over him, paying little attention to the other children. This oversolicitous behavior was not lost on the child, who actually made a very quick and uneventful recovery. When he was well again, he still got a kick out of showing off his eye patches to his friends and became a kind of hero, boasting and making up wild stories about how he had gotten his injury. At home he continued to use his "painful eye" as an excuse when he was naughty or fussy. Thus, though the period of incapacity had been short and the parents were attentive to maintaining contact with the child (covering the eyes may cause a kind of sensory deprivation), they had overdone it and let the child drag the incident out too long. The child had learned that there were considerable gains from his injury, and he made the most of it long after it had healed. His next injury might not be so "accidental"—and a pattern of injuring himself every time things weren't going to his satisfaction could be established, and even anticipated.

THE ATTENTION-GAINING BADGE

Fractures cause pain, discomfort, and varying degrees of incapacity. If you've had one, you know how much. But once the fracture is set, the cast applied, and you can get about a bit, you often don't at all mind the attention the cast attracts. It becomes something special, almost a badge rather than a mechanical device that helps in the healing process. It makes you an object of curiosity; everyone asks how you got it. Even people who don't know you look at it, and you can see them wondering what happened—perhaps an adventurous, thrilling, maybe even dangerous event had caused this fracture. You find it's not at all unpleasant to attract so much attention and conjecture. You may even begin to make up wonderful daydreams that you didn't really get it slipping on a banana peel—but by losing your balance on treacherous terrain as you approached the top of Mount Everest.

A cast is especially admired among youngsters; it becomes a romantic symbol, something to leave one's mark on, a place for graffiti. Crutches, slings, patches are other objects that attract admiration, attention, pity, sympathy, forbearance, forgiveness. So having a disability or a deformity can turn out to be as rewarding for an adult as for the five-year-old with the injured eye; and adults have the capacity for being even more ingenious about dragging out the benefits, using every means from presenting new symptoms to instituting law suits so that they can parade before juries and judges months later. And every once in a while we hear about a record jackpot being collected in the courts by an injured person.

All of us—no matter what types of injuries or illnesses we have, and no matter how seldom or frequently we are sick or disabled—find some gratification in being indisposed. Deriving such secondary gain is common and harmless—so

240

long as our self-indulgence remains within bounds. But we are in trouble if illness or injury is used to gain emotional satisfaction we should be getting through other means. We are in trouble if we let secondary gain become habitual so that we end up living off our disability. Then indeed we can forecast that we will be sick or bothered by symptoms indefinitely.

PART FIVE

New Preventive Measures

20

Using Your Emotional Alarm System

AVOIDING A THOUSAND TORTURES

To prevent disease, or to detect it in its earliest stages, is to avoid a thousand tortures. In the past, we have relied on bodily indication—bleeding, lumps, weight loss—to signal that something's going wrong with our health. But, as we have seen throughout the book, there are also psychological signs—stress, habitual ways of adaptation, denial or absence of feelings, repressed rage turned against the self, aberrations of guilt response, certain dreams, somatic identification, and blocking of adequate psychological outlets—which play a role in forecasting the possibility of physical illness. They are not intended in any sense to replace the body indicators which are so valuable. They are meant to be used *in addition* to these; they provide a new dimension to the resources of medical science for early detection of illness and prevention of serious, even fatal consequences. Furthermore, when disease does not respond even to the best medical and surgical procedures, psychological indicators may provide an answer to the failure of recovery. Learning to recognize and use these is a most effective way to safeguard our health.

PSYCHOLOGICAL SIGNS HEEDED

The earlier an illness can be detected, the more likely it can be stopped before possibly dangerous complications set in. Here's an example in which a sensible and concerned wife intervened to avert tragedy. Lowensteen, a sixty-year-old customer's man who had done only one thing all his adult life—sell stocks for commission—was fired without warning of any kind. Actually, as the market had turned bearish, his accounts had steadily shrunk. He had not, like others, pressed his customers to turn over their stocks so he could at least get something in commissions out of that. He thought his behavior a sign of honesty. Actually he was a timid person who felt inferior and always tried to be a nice guy. He was thoroughly deflated when he told his wife the bad news. She tried to console him, but his appearance troubled her. A perceptive woman, she recognized that he was in a state of emotional shock, and she worried about the consequences. In the past when things had become rough at work, he would get sick: He had had many colds and twice he had come down with painful, swollen neck glands and a lingering weakness. A definite diagnosis could not be made. It took him a long time to recover from each of these two episodes of illness. Now, although he was unaware that the new and greatest stress might make him ill again, his wife in an intuitive way was sensing this possibility.

The next day Lowensteen began to pound the pavements, but without luck. He registered at the unemployment service. Several times he thought he had a lead, but nothing ever materialized. More pounding of the pavements, more standing in line for his unemployment check. Suddenly, after several weeks of utter discouragement, his mood shifted. He became cheerful because, he said, he had decided to forget stocks and go into a brand new field. His wife was dubious, and she was more troubled than ever about him, especially because she could see that nothing had really changed. She suspected his cheerfulness was only a cover-up, that he was really as deeply discouraged as before; she didn't like this unnatural behavior, but she kept her thoughts to herself. In fact, his inadequate attempts to belittle his troubles were another signal that the strain could hurt his body.

Lowensteen couldn't get a job in any new field either, but he kept on trying to be cheerful. One night he woke up screaming. He had dreamed that an avalanche had buried him. This was still another sign that something physical could be brewing in him. The next morning while standing in line to get his unemployment check, he began to feel dizzy and almost passed out. When he got home, his alarmed wife insisted he see the family doctor. Nothing was found except some slight changes in the blood cells which the doctor wanted checked out by a specialist. He, too, was worried by Lowensteen's transparent cheerfulness and the way he was pretending that the past weeks hadn't been tough. He feared Lowensteen might be on the brink of some serious mental or physical breakdown and suggested psychotherapy. Lowensteen needed relief from the horrible tension that was there. He began a course of psychotherapy for a nominal fee at a nearby clinic. After a half-dozen visits his overall anxiety was greatly reduced. He abandoned his unrealistic plan and plugged away at getting a job once again as a customer's man, which he finally did. The blood condition which first looked like a precursor of leukemia gradually reverted to normal. The psychological signs had been heeded, thanks to his wife and his family doctor. A possibly serious illness had been averted.

PSYCHOLOGICAL SIGNS UNHEEDED

In another case a knowledge of the emotional warning signals might have led to a happier outcome. Miss Twomey had been an executive secretary in one company for many years. Now in her early fifties, living alone, she seemed reconciled to the life of a spinster. She never missed a day of work, so it was an event when Miss Twomey did not appear at her desk one Monday morning.

Actually, six months before, things had changed for her when one of the company executives died suddenly. What people did not know was that she had made up for her quiet, uneventful real life by constructing elaborate fantasies about herself and this man. It did not matter that he actually never showed the slightest interest in her in real life—in her daydreams he showered her with gifts and affection, they did exciting things together and traveled to exotic places, and she was constantly loved. Miss Twomey was shocked at his death, but it was impossible to tell anyone of her grief without also revealing the incredible fantasies on which she had been living for years. For the first week or so, she had trouble sleeping, but then she undertook to push the painful thoughts about her dead lover from her mind. She threw herself into her work and into being more generous than ever in her attention, sympathy, and advice to people at work. So Miss Twomey had compounded her problem by pretending it didn't exist, when actually she had not settled her shocked feelings at the news of her would be lover's death. Avoidance of unpleasant reality was an old pattern with her. In the past, it had helped tide her over rough situations. Now it could not; the stress would be too great and too persistent.

Most of her life she had been free of physical illness. There was one notable exception when, as a child, she had been terribly envious of her beautiful younger sister and wished her out of the way. Shortly thereafter, when the sister developed meningitis and died, Miss Twomey had suffered inwardly, convinced she had killed her. Just when it seemed she had pushed all this out of her mind, her appendix exploded and she was desperately sick. She thought her illness a fitting punishment, and this made her feel much less guilty. When she recovered, she was a different person. She wanted nothing for herself and thought only of others. However, shortly before her fantasy lover's death, she had learned that he was more than casually interested in a co-worker. Miss Twomey was so upset that for the second time in her life she wished someone dead. And for the second time in her life the person she had wished dead promptly died. The loss of her imagined lover was highly stressful; in addition her conscience was terribly disturbed; worst of all, she was trying to deny both of these things—all signs that her body might suffer from the pent-up emotion.

Even as her mind appeared less troubled, at least on the surface, Miss Twomey began to have vague abdominal cramps that came and went. The severe tension she was trying to hide was attacking her body. But she paid no attention to the cramps either. Unfortunately, she was now denying the initial symptoms of a dangerous illness. One night she dreamed she was pregnant and a monstrous man struck her swollen abdomen. She awoke in fright, sweating and breathless. The dream recurred several times the following month. She could not figure out why she was having these dreams; she had no idea that this was still another indication signaling a drastic change in her body. Nor was she aware of the other signs—the stress, the denial of feelings and symptoms, the inadequacy of her substitute relationships, the previous illness in her gut during emotional crises, the long-standing and now reactivated guilt which had been shut off. Instead of going away, the cramps became worse until that weekend, when a persistent diarrhea with reddish-looking stools frightened her into finally calling a doctor.

So that's where she was that Monday morning—in a hospital, being operated on, because X rays had shown a growth in her large bowel. It was a cancer, she was told, and there had been some spread, but the outlook wasn't so bad. What the surgeon did *not* tell her was that it was a rapidly developing cancer, and if only it had been picked up a few months before, the prognosis would have been much better.

This case is striking because the loss which precipitated the illness was imaginary. Even though there never *had* been a relationship between Miss Twomey and the executive, and their intimacy had existed only in her fantasies, to her it had been real all these years. And the loss was just as real as if the whole affair had actually taken place. And because it was so, her reaction had been extreme.

PSYCHOLOGICAL SIGNS MISSED

While psychotherapy helped Lowensteen, it is not a panacea. Some psychotherapists are not aware that psychological manifestations herald more than emotional disturbance. Consider Rennie who began his studies in philosophy at age twelve. He was encouraged by his father, a brute of a man whose liver disease had almost killed him after a climactic drinking bout. His mother, troubled by a chronic bladder condition, didn't like her son's philosophic bent and wanted him to become a doctor. By the time Rennie had graduated from high school, he was thoroughly confused. First, he undertook a major in philosophy at college, but then shifted to get his bachelor's degree in science; then he returned to his original plans, grew restless, and went back to graduate studies in science. Unable to decide upon a career, he started psychotherapy. Shortly afterward, he met a girl and slept with her—the first time for him. Although he had twinges of guilt about it, the relationship continued until she announced she was pregnant. Rennie was terrified and began to make inquiries about abortion. Then a severe sore throat laid him up. Although he had fever, he wouldn't let a doctor be called. After a few days Rennie got out of bed, shaky and weak, and tried to get back into the swing of things. When he saw his girl friend and she informed him that she wasn't pregnant after all, he suddenly struck her in the face. He had never hit a girl before, and he was overwhelmed by feelings of self-recrimination. When she had first told him he had impregnated her, he had had secret thoughts which made him feel triumphantly that he was a man. Now he felt terribly let down. He was ashamed to mention it in therapy, and after a few days his mind blanked on the whole thing. Instead he talked a lot about his past. Ever since he'd been a kid, he had had doubts about his masculinity. His father's awesome size made him feel like a nothing in those days. Rennie's childhood bedwetting which continued for several years reinforced his lack of confidence in himself. Later, he had brief bouts of nonspecific prostatitis, but he failed to note that they occurred when he was under unusual tension.

The therapist was well aware that Rennie had been subjected to severe emotional stresses, but he concentrated only on the psychological problems, not on any possible physical effects. So even though Rennie complained of exhaustion and a little burning on urination, the therapist did not fit all the pieces together to predict possible illness.

One night shortly thereafter, Rennie couldn't sleep; he felt terrible. Yet his misery was strangely exciting in a sexual way, and he began to masturbate—and was stunned to experience great pain. The next morning when he tried to urinate he screamed; it hurt so much he felt he had been cut. At the infirmary an ominous diagnosis was made: a severe infection of the kidneys—acute glomerulonephritis. The doctors told him it had all probably started with that bad sore throat some weeks before, which he had neglected. Dangerous strep germs had invaded his kidneys, causing the havoc. His therapist had been too preoccupied with Rennie's emotional problems and not sufficiently familiar with the significance of the psychological warning of likely physical changes.

THE EARLIEST DETECTION OF
CANCER

The outcome was different for Mrs. Massey, a suburban housewife with time on her hands. The children were off at school. Her husband's medical practice made him often unavailable for companionship, and they had gradually drifted apart. Just like her own parents. They had been an unhappy couple and she, an only child, had been right in the middle. Very early she had discovered that if she got sick, that would bring the quarreling to an end temporarily. By the time she was fourteen, she had had all the childhood illnesses, her tonsils and appendix had been removed, and she had an anemia that persisted for several years. When she was in college, her parents were finally divorced. It was then that she suddenly decided to marry a promising young internist.

For some years afterward she was quite free of illness. She had tried to be a good mother to her own two daughters, and she was stunned and bewildered at the news that her elder daughter had been arrested in a drug raid. In the horrible weeks that followed, even though her daughter finally got off with a suspended sentence, Mrs. Massey was faced with trying to figure it all out. Where had things gone wrong? What was her part in this mess? Her husband, far from providing consolation, accused her of having spoiled the kids. It was no secret that his lack of concern for her was owing to his involvement with another woman. All of this falling apart of her life confused her. She had never felt so tight and taut before.

Months passed and she had managed to put out of her mind any thoughts of her husband's affair or of their wayward daughter. Mrs. Massey seemed outwardly quite calm, even serene. But she could not continue to deceive herself; she was inwardly as tense as ever, and she felt she was apt to become ill under the strain, just as she had so often in childhood. No physical symptoms yet, but it was time to talk to someone. She made an appointment to see her internist. He listened attentively as she spoke about her recent troubles and persistent tension. Despite the absence of any distinct physical symptoms, he did a careful examination. He took somewhat longer than usual palpating her breasts. She had not noticed any difference or change in them. Once more, he felt the area near her right nipple. There it was, an olive-sized lump not visible but detectable by palpation. Her doctor advised an immediate surgical consultation, which in turn confirmed the need for quick exploration of the area.

She was operated on the next day. It was a small tumor. A frozen section done and examined right after the lump had been removed revealed just a few nests of cancer cells. Very, very early. No spread. As a routine preventive measure the breast was removed, but the outlook was excellent. The disease had really been caught in time. Mrs. Massey had had no sophisticated knowledge of psychological clues in forecasting illness, but her recollection of how emotion had wracked her body in the past and her intuition both served her well. In fact, they probably saved her life.

Most cancers have a good outlook for recovery or long-lasting improvement, *if* they are detected early enough. The American Cancer Society has listed the physical warning signs of this disease. If we heed them and immediately get medical advice, a favorable outcome is likely. However, it is possible to go further in combating cancer by also using the psychological clues I have discussed. Then, the disease might be prevented from developing altogether. Even if cancer has already begun, but is at a stage where no clear-cut physical signs are present, psychological clues can help detect its presence, possibly even its location.

Let me illustrate step-by-step how this can work.

Craig, 45 years old, came to see me after his wife had left him. He was obviously depressed. In the past he had dealt with his marital troubles by using the psychological mechanism which in psychiatry is called denial. He had simply acted as if nothing was wrong. This time his wife's actions were so extreme he could no longer deny them, and he felt very lonely and sad. Under his self-assured exterior was a basic emotional dependence on other people, and this came to the fore when his marriage broke up.

Stress, denial which breaks down, and activated emotional dependency can lead to many outcomes. Craig could remain in a depression or recover from it. His use of denial could become effective again. The veneer of self-confidence could be restored. All this might happen without any treatment but under favorable life circumstances such as a new and meaningful close relationship with another person. Moreover, any guilt feelings he had might run only a limited course and the depression would then subside.

If none of these circumstances favored him, his sadness might continue, deepen, and require some form of treatment: chemotherapy, psychotherapy, or both. However, should he be unable to drain off his tensions psychologically, then the depression would be replaced by some body disturbance. There were already psychological clues which pointed to this possibility.

I discussed all this with him and recommended some short-term therapy if he didn't feel better in a few weeks. Six months later he again asked for a consultation. He had had no treatment of any kind in the interim. The divorce had gone through and curiously his depression seemed to subside. He had met an attractive younger woman who began to mother him.

Why had he come to see me again? He had been experiencing a vague sense of generalized tension ever since he had heard that his father was ill. At first, he didn't know the nature of the sickness, only that his father had been losing weight. He traveled several thousand miles to see his father and the visit had "unnerved" him. He felt that his mother was selfishly absorbed in herself and didn't care what happened to her husband.

Not once did the patient show any anger or much of any emotion at all. He spoke in a bland tone of voice. Yet it was evident from the content of his remarks that he was furious at his mother's attitude.

He later learned that his father was getting chemical treatments. The doctors had declared his condition inoperable. He had cancer of the colon. After telling me this Craig had a burst of recollections about wanting to emulate and beat his father's accomplishments as a sportsman. But he described himself as a "poor imitation."

Shortly after his return from his visit to his father, Craig began to experience "butterflies" in his stomach. It was a sensation he could not recall ever having had before. In fact, he had insisted he always had been well. Actually, he had had frequent minor episodes of indigestion, which he passed off as "nothing."

How did I assess his situation on this occasion? A warm mothering figure had entered the picture, ordinarily a mitigating psychological factor. But this was countered by new stresses: a gravely ill father with whom he had competed and identified in the past, and the continuing selfishness of his mother. Then there were absence of anger, evidence that denial was again becoming inadequate as a psychological defense, and a persistent *new* physical sensation.

I told Craig that it was imperative for him to get a thorough physical checkup at once. But he delayed doing so. Some weeks later he had "stomach flu"—so it was diagnosed by his physician and reported to me. After "recovering" from his "flu," he called me on the telephone to say he was feeling much better and had decided to remarry.

A month went by and Craig then called me for still another consultation, saying he was tense again. He told me that after each of his previous visits to me he had felt calmer and hoped that this would happen again. He had been having troublesome dreams. Several times he dreamed that he was disintegrating, that the middle part of his body was disappearing. I noted his almost dull, controlled mechanical speech. His eyes were fixed on me during the entire interview. The marriage? He couldn't satisfy his new wife sexually. He had lost the urge. He had also begun to have episodes of nausea, but he called it "more of the same stuff I've always had."

I explored his resistance to having a physical checkup. He was afraid of a "bad diagnosis," of a disfiguring operation, of not being able to continue to be manly and becoming a chronic invalid. I was able to reduce his anxiety and to reinforce his motivation for living. This time he did go for a complete physical examination. The findings were not clear cut. X rays showed only an ill-defined suspicious area in the stomach. I discussed my own specific psychological findings with his other doctors who had also noted Craig's controlled tension. We agreed that an exploratory operation was indicated. A small mass was found in the stomach —and it was very early cancer. There was no spread of the disease. The outlook was for complete recovery.

The psychological clues had *added* up in such a way that they imperatively indicated the need for immediate medical action. If there had been any delay, the outcome might well have been different.

Cancer is such a treacherous disease because often it begins without any noticeable signs or symptoms. During such very early stages, the most advanced instrumentation and lab tests may not pick up any evidence that the cancerous process has started. Even when physical signs begin to appear, they are not always clear, so they are disregarded by the patient; or else they are so puzzling to the doctor that he has difficulty making a certain diagnosis. But as we have seen there are also psychological clues to the development of cancer. The trouble has been that until recently the relationship between emotion and the start of a cancer has been formulated in such vague and simplistic terms that practical application of the findings to make diagnoses has been disappointing. The suggestion that there is a "cancer personality" is really of little use. It is an attempt to package a few personality traits which supposedly provide a quick answer as to who is likely to develop the disease. The trouble is that the general characteristics for the "cancer personality" can be found in people who come down with other physical or emotional illnesses. The same is true of "coronary personality," "ulcer personality," and so on.

At this stage in the development of our knowledge about mind-body relationships, I have found the psychological clues described throughout the book to be of practical use in predicting and detecting illness. These signs also signal the likely recurrence of cancer or any other disease in which relapses might be expected, such as coronary thrombosis, arthritis, ulcer. In addition, when illness does not respond to the best medical or surgical procedures, the psychological clues may provide an answer to the puzzling question of why recovery is not taking place. But—as I have already stated—using your emotional alarm system in all these situations is not intended to replace, but to supplement, physical indications.

LITTLE CONSIDERED PREVENTIVE MEASURES

Even today, when psychology and psychiatry have contributed to our knowledge of emotion—both external *and* internal—people still deal with it in an erratic way as a factor in physical illness—if they deal with it at all. That includes the nonpsychiatrically trained doctor who sees the bulk of psychological disorders, even as they are developing and possibly affecting our susceptibility to bodily disturbances. Unfortunately, many physicians are not yet familiar with the emotional signs (other than stress) which warn of such sickness. True, if you have an obvious major mental disturbance, you probably will be referred to a psychiatrist. But for the most part, many doctors will examine and treat you on a purely physical basis. In many annual checkups, meticulous attention is paid to physical signs, X rays, and laboratory tests, but no inquiry is made about psychological indication of possible bodily disorders. Of course, if your doctor is understanding and genuinely interested in you as a person, he will take the time to talk to you about your emotional problems. This is a good start, because verbal communication between patient and doctor is absolutely necessary for a comprehensive understanding of illness, its prevention, its diagnosis, and treatment. But not just any verbal communication! Your family doctor, well meaning as he may be, needs to have not only some understanding of human behavior but also an awareness of what psychological signs indicate that physical illness is impending or that complications may develop. Then he can institute preventive measures designed to provide reassurance, allow you to let off some steam, and alleviate troublesome symptoms—and if your indisposition is minor, this may be all you need.

But, suppose you have been under considerable stress and it doesn't seem to be abating. It may trigger a physical illness—perhaps a serious one. If at all feasible, you might consider having some short-term preventive psychotherapy. I don't mean a psychoanalysis, but some interviews at a community clinic or discussions about your immediate emotional problems with a person trained to deal with them, so that you can be helped to rid yourself of tension—and with it the likelihood of a breakdown. Sometimes there is a relatively long interval between the time the manifestations of a change in your psychological state are noticeable and the appearance of physical illness. Six months or more may elapse. Attention to all the psychological clues we have mentioned is especially important during this interim.

Unrelieved emotional upset manifested by these signs over such a long period is very likely indeed to end in bodily disease. If you are already severely ill physically, it can be dangerous to ignore the impact that your unconscious is having on your body. Crippling or fatal consequences can be avoided if your doctor notes any accompanying emotional warning signals, understands their meaning, and institutes whatever additional measures are indicated.

Psychoanalysis has taught us a lot about how our emotions affect our illnesses. But this does not mean you have to have an analysis yourself to benefit from the application of its theories. Analysis is costly, time-consuming, not indicated or successful in certain disorders or individuals, and you wouldn't always be able to find the proper trained person even if the treatment were recommended. Actually it is available or indicated for only a small fraction of the emotionally sick and only in highly selected instances for those physically ill. But to benefit from the *findings* of psychoanalysis is something within the reach of us all. The *applications* of its basic theory are invaluable in the following: (1) understanding psychological signs of impending physical illness and their use in prevention of disease; (2) predicting our reactions to medical or surgical treatment; (3) foreseeing how our emotions will influence the course of disease, convalescence, and recovery—and how these are best dealt with to avoid complications. I have tried in previous chapters to deal with all these aspects in some detail.

THE IMPORTANCE OF MOTIVATION

Let me now add a clue that is of great assistance in forecasting whether or not preventive methods (or other treatment) will be effective. That is our motivation to be well. For instance, how can coronary thrombosis best be prevented, using an approach which includes both physical *and* emotional factors? Here's what some researchers suggest. (1) Counter stress and excessive stimulation of the nervous system and adrenal cortex by a change to a more relaxed environment, increased physical activity, weight reduction, giving up tobacco, and starting psychotherapy. (2) Slow down development of atherosclerosis (which narrows the coronary arteries and diminishes the vital supply of blood to the heart) by avoiding cholesterol-rich foods, and control any high blood pressure or diabetes by treatment. Now, all this is well and good—it's easy to outline. But suppose you're emotionally resistive to all these recommendations, not motivated to follow them consistently, whether it's giving up smoking, engaging in more physical activity, going on a strict diet, taking medicines, getting psychotherapy, and so on. What then? There is a widespread, naive belief that if the doctor (or other health professional) recommends one or another course of treatment, we will automatically follow this advice. That isn't necessarily so. Powerful emotional forces in us may interfere: denial, which influences us to think that nothing is wrong and that we don't need any medical, surgical, or psychiatric help; fright, which makes us picture treatment as worse than whatever is wrong with our bodies; suspiciousness, which leads us to question unduly the integrity of those caring for us, the medicines we are using, and the course of treatment outlined for us; self-destructiveness, which will interfere in many ways with our sticking to the prescribed regimen and thereby keep us from benefiting from it. Usually, it's only when our suffering transcends all these that we are motivated to get help and follow it through. It has been suggested that in every one of us there are powerful biological forces that impel us in the direction of health, of balanced psychological and physical functioning. There are also references to the "will to live" or to "strong self-preservative drives" as factors, not yet specifically defined, which are closely related to motivation. So for physical and psychological preventive measures against illness to have any chance of success, our motivation for carrying these out has to be assessed and whenever necessary, strengthened. In the past that has rarely been done.

Whatever the age group, prevention of illness, its early detection, and reduction of complications are basic goals toward which we continue to move. Now that more well-defined psychological clues are available which help us to predict physical disease and unfavorable outcomes, it is hoped that progress in this direction will be quickened. However, it is essential that not only health professionals, but also the lay public, be familiar with these new warnings of when to be on the lookout for illness.